MORE PRAISE FOR
Quick and Easy Low-Cal Vegan Comfort Food

"With *Quick and Easy Low-Cal Vegan Comfort Food* Alicia C. Simpson combines a sensible approach to a whole-foods vegan diet with delicious down-home recipes like Sweet Potato Soufflé, Breakfast Biscuit Sandwich, and Butter Rum Pound Cake. Healthy eating never tasted so good!" —**Robin Robertson**, best-selling author of *Quick-Fix Vegan*, *Vegan on the Cheap*, and *Vegan Fire & Spice*

"Alicia's enticing recipes are nutrient-rich, flavor-packed, and built from familiar, whole ingredients, and her delightful descriptions make you feel like she's in the kitchen with you preparing delicious, sensible meals."
  —**Colleen Patrick-Goudreau**, best-selling author of *Color Me Vegan*, *Vegan's Daily Companion*, and *The 30-Day Vegan Challenge*

"Alicia has really outdone herself with this book. Finally we can have decadent soul food without the calories or fat. Many of Alicia's recipes are made without oil and using wholesome, fresh ingredients. I highly recommend this book!"
  —**Lindsay S. Nixon**, author of *The Happy Herbivore Cookbook* and *Everyday Happy Herbivore*

"This book is a must-have for anyone (vegan or not!) who is looking to get rid of excess calories and keep all of the fun and flavor in comfort food favorites. Alicia shows us how to control portions while discussing the nutritional science from a vegan point of view in a book that is thoughtfully laid out and fun to read." —**Joni Marie Newman**, coauthor of *The Complete Guide to Vegan Food Substitutions*

"Forget having to drop the fun and flavor from your meals in order to make them figure-friendly, because Alicia's *Quick & Easy Low-Cal Vegan Comfort Food* will have you dreaming of lower-calorie vegan Cheese Fries, Chorizo Breakfast Quesadillas, and Strawberry Cheesecake Ice Cream, and devouring them too!"
  —**Celine Steen**, coauthor of *Hearty Vegan Meals for Monster Appetites*

"From Baked Hush Puppies and Vegetable Noodle Soup to Chickpea Cacciatore and Lemongrass Soda, Alicia has some amazing recipes in store for you. Welcome to the new world of good-for-you comfort food!" —**Kathy Hester**, author of *The Vegan Slow Cooker*

THE EXPERIMENT

BECAUSE EVERY BOOK IS A TEST OF NEW IDEAS

Also by Alicia C. Simpson

Quick and Easy Vegan Comfort Food:
65 Everyday Meal Ideas for Breakfast, Lunch and Dinner
with Over 150 Great-Tasting, Down-Home Recipes

Quick and Easy Vegan Celebrations:
150 Great-Tasting Recipes Plus Festive Menus
for Vegantastic Holidays and Get-Togethers
All Through the Year

QUICK AND EASY

LOW-CAL
Vegan Comfort Food

150 DOWN-HOME RECIPES

PACKED WITH FLAVOR,

NOT CALORIES

Alicia C. Simpson

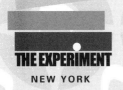

THE EXPERIMENT

NEW YORK

Quick and Easy Low-Cal Vegan Comfort Food: *150 Down-Home Recipes Packed with Flavor, Not Calories*

The Experiment
260 Fifth Avenue, Suite 3 South
New York, NY 10001-6408
www.theexperimentpublishing.com

This book contains the opinions and ideas of its author. It is intended to provide helpful and informative material on the subjects addressed in the book. It is sold with the understanding that the author and publisher are not engaged in rendering medical, health, or any other kind of personal professional services in the book. The author and publisher specifically disclaim all responsibility for any liability, loss, or risk—personal or otherwise—that is incurred as a consequence, directly or indirectly, of the use and application of any of the contents of this book.

The Experiment's books are available at special discounts when purchased in bulk for premiums and sales promotions as well as for fundraising or educational use. For details, contact us at info@theexperimentpublishing.com.

Library of Congress Cataloging-in-Publication Data
Simpson, Alicia C.
Quick and easy low-cal vegan comfort food : 150 down-home recipes packed
with flavor, not calories / Alicia C. Simpson.
p. cm.
Includes index.
ISBN 978-1-61519-042-3 (pbk.)—ISBN 1-61519-042-2 (pbk.)—ISBN
978-1-61519-142-0 (ebook)—ISBN 1-61519-142-9 (ebook) 1. Vegan cooking.
2. Comfort food. 3. Low-calorie diet—Recipes. I. Title.
TX837.S497 2011
641.5'636—dc23
2011043502

ISBN: 978-1-61519-042-3
Ebook ISBN: 978-1-61519-142-0

Cover design by Susi Oberhelman
Cover photographs © Sara Lynn Paige, featuring Seitan Cheesesteak (page 193) and oven-baked fries from
    Cheese Fries (page 120)
Author photograph by Kelly Donovan
Text design by Pauline Neuwirth, Neuwirth & Associates, Inc.

Manufactured in the United States of America
Distributed by Workman Publishing Company, Inc.
Distributed simultaneously in Canada by Thomas Allen and Son Ltd.

First published May 2012
10 9 8 7 6 5 4 3 2 1

To my parents John and Linda Simpson.

You are two of the most supportive, loving, and giving people

I have ever been blessed to know. You are what love is.

Contents

Note: 📷 indicates that the recipe is pictured in the photo insert.

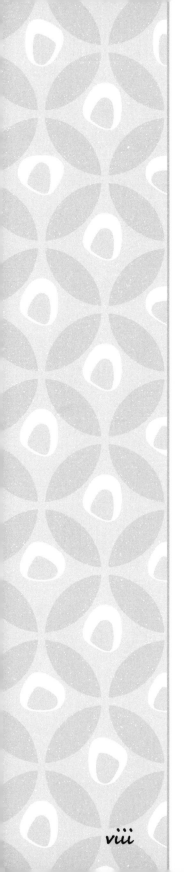

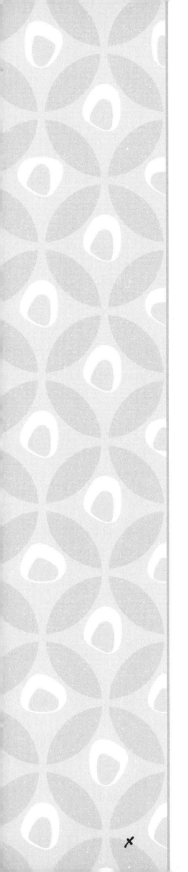

The Main Event   155

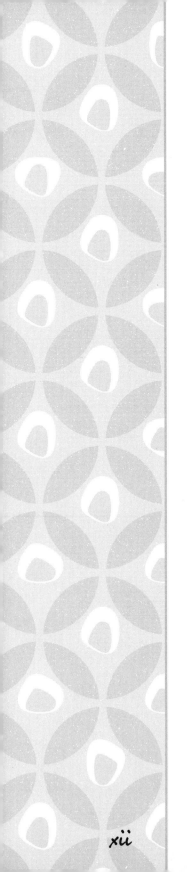

QUICK AND EASY

LOW-CAL
Vegan Comfort Food

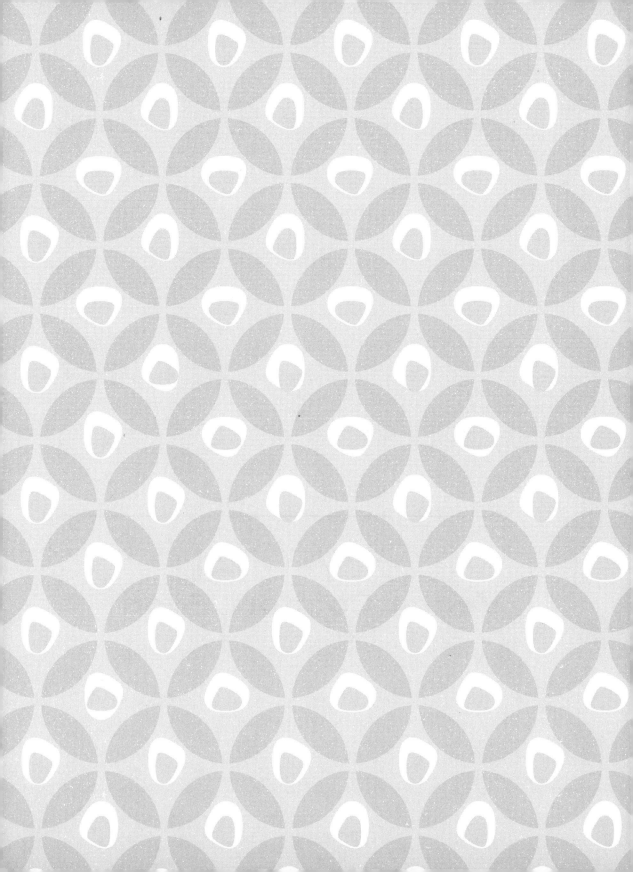

Low-Calorie, Full Flavor

IT'S CONFESSION TIME. I'm not your typical low-calorie, low-fat health nut. My policy has always been simply to eat the foods I love, exercise daily, and keep a positive attitude. When I set out to write this book, my philosophy on food stayed the same. Although the recipes in this book are low-calorie, none of them were designed specifically to be low-calorie (except for Fettucine Slim-Fredo, page 158, by popular request). When I developed these recipes, I was cooking the way I've always cooked: using full-fat oils, real sugar, and nothing "diet." *Low-Calorie Vegan Comfort Food* isn't about depriving yourself—it's about conscious eating. In this book I give you the tools you need to be alert to calorie intake and portion sizes so you can eat plenty of real food while maintaining or losing weight, as you choose.One of the biggest problems with diets is that they have so many restrictions: low carb, low fat, high protein—the list goes on and on. When it comes right down to it, weight loss is as simple as eating about 100 fewer calories a day than you typically would and getting out there and moving around a little bit more every day. There's no magic formula; it's really just that simple. Thankfully, veganism makes this so much easier, because fruit, vegetables, grains, nuts, seeds, and legumes are all naturally rich in vitamins, minerals, and protein which are typically lower in fat than animal products. So congratulations! Your decision to eat a plant-based vegan diet has already put you on the right road towards a better you. However, where many vegans go wrong is falling into the "junk food vegan" trap, snacking on cookies, cupcakes, pies, vegan candy bars, and processed foods all day. Being vegan doesn't automatically equal great health and a healthy body weight, but being what I

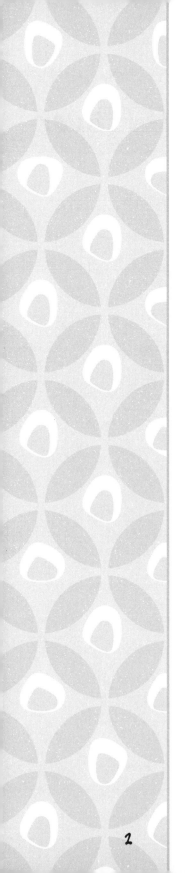

call a "whole foods vegan" will help put you on the right track. By "whole foods vegan," I don't mean vegans who shop at the popular health food chain by the same name, but vegans who eat a wholesome diet made up of generous servings of nutrient-rich whole grains, fruits, vegetables, legumes, nuts, and seeds—not a diet made up of nutrient-poor junk foods.

Not to worry, there is still room in your life for your favorite sweet treats. This book has a chapter dedicated to Sinful Sweets (page 199), and it is filled with recipes for donuts, ice creams, cakes, and cupcakes. Actually, it is surprising how few calories are in many desserts. The real problem arises when we eat three cupcakes instead of one, or two cups of ice cream instead of a half-cup serving. This won't be a problem for you, though, because this book will teach you how to use proper serving sizes to create satisfying meals with real food and work in your favorite desserts, too, without a single calorie more than you need.

Redefining Comfort Food

FOOD IS SO many things: it's pleasurable, it brings us together, it reminds us of home, it brings back fond memories of people we love and places we've been. For vegans, it's an outward expression of our ethical beliefs. Often, however, we forget the role that food plays in *physical* nourishment. We forget that everything we put in our mouths does serve a purpose. That our hearts need fat to function, our brains need sugar for sustenance, our muscles need protein to repair themselves, and every reaction that happens in our body on the tiniest molecular level requires a careful balance of vitamins, minerals, proteins, carbohydrates, and fats to occur. If you've ever thumbed through my first two books *Quick and Easy Vegan Comfort Food* and *Quick and Easy Vegan Celebrations* then you already know that I'm a Caliornia girl through and through. To that end, Mexican food is what I consider comfort food. Now that I live in Georgia if I told someone I was having a comfort food dinner and served my traditional fare of tacos, enchiladas, Mexican Rice (page 115), Refried Beans (page 112), and Queso Dip (page 100) with homemade Baked Tortilla Chips (page 98) they would look at me like I had sprouted a third eye from my elbow. Here in Georgia, comfort food is macaroni and cheese, collard greens, candied yams, and anything fried.

Comfort food means something different to everyone. It's the food that takes you back home in one bite. There might be some food in this book that strikes you as being great food but not necessarily comfort food—like Millet Tabbouleh (page 138), Amaranth-Quinoa Salad (page 139), and Indian-Spiced Chickpeas (page 187)—but it's important to remember that the definition of comfort food changes from region to region and person to

person. Trying dishes that are slightly outside your comfort zone might actually bring you closer to redefining comfort food for yourself and adding a whole new reptoire of dishes to your weekly menu. The goal of this book is to make you smile with every bite of vegan comfort food—without tipping the scales.

Move Your Butt!

WHETHER YOUR GOAL is to lose weight or just to live a healthier life, exercising is essential. Our bodies are engineered for motion, and the sedentary lifestyle so common now is quite new in the history of humans. Just one generation ago, walking to and from work and school and, very literally, "running" errands were commonplace. Now our fast-paced, car-dependent lifestyles are less and less conducive to the near-constant motion our bodies are designed for. We are often stuck sitting all day at a desk then on long commutes to and from work. Not only that but we often live too far from the stores we patronize to walk. Our concept of exercise has changed, too. When my parents were growing up in the 1950s and '60s you could hardly find a gym anywhere. There was no need for one; the world was your gymnasium. Now it sometimes seems as if the gym is the only place to get good-quality exercise. Luckily, this couldn't be further from the truth.

The world is still your gymnasium, no matter where you live. You don't have to run a 5K or be able to lift a hundred pounds to be physically fit. The simple act of taking a brisk thirty-minute walk every day is fantastic. So is taking the stairs at work, both up and down. You can do something as simple as not driving around the parking lot for ten minutes to find the space closest to the door; instead, parking in the back and taking a leisurely walk up. Did you lose the remote control for your television for the umpteenth time? Instead of spending fifteen minutes looking for it, why not just walk up to the TV and change the channel like in the old days? Every opportunity you have to move your butt, take it!

Learn the Language

THE WORLD OF low-calorie or "diet" food is a daunting one. Even the term "low-calorie" is an ambiguous one. What does *low-calorie* really mean? What does *low-fat* mean? Should you be counting calories? What about carbs? And how important is protein? The market is flooded with so many fad diet books it's hard to tell which is based in legitimate science and which is just another marketing scheme. From time to time, people have even tried to push a vegan lifestyle into the "diet" category, but as any longtime vegan will tell you, going vegan does not guarantee weight loss. In fact, within the first six months of going vegan I gained ten pounds and was at my highest weight ever! Then I became a whole food vegan, eating wholesome, unprocessed foods, not many sweets, and making sure that I had every food group represented at each meal. And make no mistake, meat is not a stand-alone food group, and neither is dairy. In fact in the recent 2011 food guidelines dairy has been taken off the plate all together, literally. Switching to whole foods was all it took: the weight came off, and I'm happy to report it hasn't come back.

LOW-FAT AND LOW-CALORIE

The terms *low-calorie* and *low-fat* are strictly regulated by the Food and Drug Administration (FDA) when they appear on the labels of commercial foods. Anything with 40 calories or less per serving is considered low-calorie, and anything with under 3 grams of fat per serving is low-fat. These are useful guidelines that keep cookie manufacturers from labeling their products low-calorie, but for the practical purposes of planning an entire, multicomponent meal that includes a rich protein source, vegetables, fruit, and whole grains, the guidelines don't really apply. A 40-calorie meal is clearly not enough to eat, and a 40-calorie serving of twelve different items may be too much. As a general rule, keeping meals and major meal components under 350 calories, as I've done in this book, will help you maintain a diet that works toward almost any weight goal, whether it be to gain weight, lose weight, or maintain your weight. And it will make life much simpler.

SERVING SIZE

Serving sizes vary for just about everything you put in your mouth, so it's no wonder that most people are confused about what a real serving size is. You've probably heard that portion sizes in the Standard American Diet have gotten way out of control, but how do you turn down a platter full of food when it's sitting right there in front of you, begging to be eaten?

Serving sizes can get complicated fast. Every food has its own recommended serving size, and some have several! The United States Department of Agriculture (USDA) has one set of serving sizes on which they base their public health campaigns, like the 2011 My Plate model. Manufacturers have their own agendas, and they use their own arbitrary numbers to create serving sizes. The best thing you can do as a consumer is to learn what a serving size is for *yourself*; then you will know how to portion out any meal that's in front of you and how to read and understand labels to learn what is in the packaged foods you buy and how much of it you should eat. The following serving sizes are good guidelines to start with.

TYPICAL SERVING SIZES

Grains
½ cup cooked pasta, rice, or corn
1 cup cereal
1 slice of bread
½ cup cooked cereal (oatmeal, Cream of Wheat, grits, etc.)
One 4-inch pancake (1½ ounces)

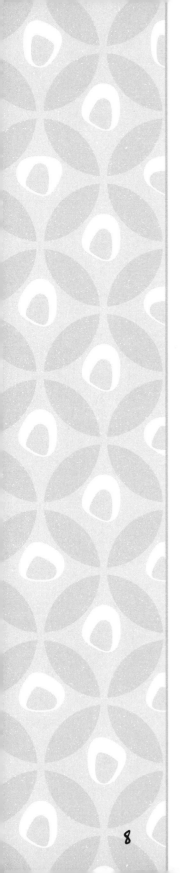

Half of a 3-inch bagel (1 ounce)
Half of an English muffin
Half of a large (9-inch) tortilla
Half of a hamburger bun

Vegetables

1 cup cooked green vegetables
2 cups raw green vegetables
12 baby carrots (about 1 cup)
¾ cup vegetable juice
1 small baked potato (2¼ ounces)
½ cup French fries (1 ounce)

Fruits

1 medium fruit
½ cup cooked, canned, or chopped fruit
¾ cup fruit juice
1 cup berries

Proteins

½ cup cooked beans, peas, or lentils
3 ounces tofu
2 tablespoons peanut butter
¼ cup almonds or shelled pistachios
⅓ cup other nuts
2 tablespoons hummus

As you get used to portioning your food properly, you will start to do it without thinking. One of the simplest ways to create a perfectly portioned meal is using the "plate method," in which half of your plate contains fruits and vegetables, one quarter is protein foods, and one quarter is grains or starches. Just remember, this is for a standard 9-inch plate that is not overflowing at the rim and piled high!

In this book I try to simplify things by dividing everything into serving sizes for you. For example, you might look at a pot of Ole-Fashioned Chili Beans (page 169) and wonder "How in the world am I supposed to know what a serving is?" Easy! Divide the pot of beans evenly among six serving dishes or small containers, and there you have it—six servings. Refrigerate any servings that don't get eaten at the meal. Do this for everything in this book. As soon as you make it, divide it up into the number of servings stated for the recipe and you're good to go. Single servings of all the recipes in this book are under 350 calories, most of them are under 250 calories, and even more hover near 150 calories or less. But even at such low numbers the calories can add up quick if you don't pay attention to how much you are eating.

COUNTING CALORIES

Truthfully, I hate counting calories. I think it is just about the most laborious, awful, no good, terrible task that has ever been invented. The only time I came close to counting calories was while I was pregnant with my daughter (which was, coincidentally, while I was writing this book). Even then I used an app so I wouldn't have to actually count a thing. That's why in this book I count calories for you. All you have to do is pay attention to your serving size; the calorie count is right there at the end of every recipe, along with information on protein, fat, sodium, and more. Once you determine what your daily calorie intake should be, you can simply enjoy eating, mixing and matching single servings of these meals and snacks throughout the day, until you've reached it.

Nearly all serving sizes and recommended daily allowances, from those on food labels to the USDA food guidelines, are based on a 2,000-calorie diet. In actual reality, that is a lot more calories than the average person needs. The only way to precisely assess how many calories you need to eat in a day is through a series of really expensive tests. For practical purposes, dietitians use several simpler, less expensive tools including the Mifflin-St. Jeor equation to calculate daily calorie needs.

The Mifflin-St. Jeor equation is done in the metric system, so to use it you'll need to convert your height and weight into metric units first. Don't panic—I'll walk you through it. To convert your weight into kilograms, simply divide your weight in pounds by 2.2 (weight in pounds ÷ 2.2 = _____ kilograms). Next, convert your height into centimeters by multiplying your height in inches by 2.54 (height in inches × 2.54 = _____ centimeters). Now you can plug these values into the first part of the Mifflin-St. Jeor equation (don't worry, there will only be two parts!).

Male: (10 × weight) + (6.25 × height) – (5 × age) + 5

(_____) + (_____) – (_____) + 5 = _____

Female: (10 × weight) + (6.25 × height) – (5 × age) – 161

(_____) + (_____) – (_____) – 161 = _____

Once you have this part of the equation figured out, multiply the number you get by one of the following numbers, which are based on your activity level. In this part of the equation many people tend to overestimate how much they actually exercise. Most people are sedentary to lightly active. If you calculate your caloric needs and find yourself gaining weight instead of losing or maintaining it, then you've probably overestimated how much you actually exercise.

1.200 = sedentary (little or no exercise)

1.375 = lightly active (light exercise/sports 1–3 days/week)

1.550 = moderately active (moderate exercise/sports 3–5 days/week)

1.725 = very active (hard exercise/sports 6–7 days a week)

1.900 = extra active (very hard exercise/sports and physical job)

Calculating the equation is pretty easy. Here's an example of a twenty-eight-year-old woman who is 5 feet 6 inches tall (66 inches × 2.54 = 167.64 centimeters) and weighs 130 pounds (130 pounds ÷ 2.2 = 59.1 kilograms) and has a desk job but tries to walk a couple times a week.

(10 x 59.1 kg) + (6.25 x 167.64 cm) – (5 x 28) – 161

(591) + (1,047.75) – (140) – 161

= 1337.75 x 1.200 (little or no exercise)

= 1,605 estimated daily calories to maintain weight

Keep in mind this is just a rough estimate. Some people cling to these numbers like they are gospel, but it isn't necessary to be fanatical about the number. It's simply a guide, a good place to start when creating weight loss, gain, or maintenance goals for yourself. Remember, this whole process should be low pressure and low stress. To get the best idea how to create a diet plan based on your estimated caloric needs, seek out a registered dietitian who specializes in vegan or vegetarian diets to help guide you.

NUTRIENT DENSITY

If you watch one or more of the many doctor-hosted television shows popping up on the air these days, you've probably heard the term "nutrient dense" tossed around a time or two. It's the foundation of good nutrition, but what does it mean? A nutrient-dense food, in the simplest sense, is just a food that is rich in nutrients. So instead of nutrient *dense*, think nutrient *rich*.

PROTEIN

There's no doubt about it. The American public is protein obsessed. We will forgo eating fruits, vegetables, nuts and seeds, and healthy whole grains to make sure that we have an abundant amount of protein in our diet. But is it really necessary, or even beneficial, to go overboard on protein? No. The average American consumes over three times the amount of protein he or she needs daily, and the average vegetarian American consumes over two times the necessary daily amount of protein.

When I first started working on my masters in nutrition I recall being one of those protein-obsessed individuals, until I was required to record everything I ate for a week and then analyze my nutrient intake. I was stunned to see that, on average, I was consuming nearly four times as much protein as I needed in a day—and that was on a vegan diet. I had minimized the amount of fruit and vegetables I was eating and replaced them with super protein-rich foods. I was eating soy-based foods, nuts, seeds, or beans at every single meal and every snack. As a result I wasn't getting all the vitamins and minerals I needed, outside of iron and calcium, because I was

completely neglecting the other very important, nutrient-rich food groups.

This is what so many Americans do every day, despite guidelines that tell us to eat differently. In fact, throughout the many evolutions of the USDA guidelines—from the food guide to the food pyramid to today's My Plate method—protein foods (including meats, legumes, nuts, and seeds) have always been one of the smallest parts of a healthy diet, while fruits, vegetables, and whole grains have always been the most important groups. The USDA Recommended Daily Allowance for protein is 0.8 grams per kilogram of body weight. So, a person who weighs 140 pounds (63.63 kg) would need about 51 grams of protein a day. However, it's important to remember when calculating your protein needs that, if you are overweight or obese that you should use your *recommended body weight,* not your current body weight, to calculate protein needs. Your protein needs are based on the amount of protein your body requires for muscle repair and biological functions and not based on any excess body fat. If you don't want to be bothered with doing any calculations—this isn't math class, after all—the Centers for Disease Control (CDC) make it simple by recommending an average of 46 grams of protein a day for women and 56 grams a day for men. If you stick with these, you really can't go wrong.

FAT

Unless you are trying to reverse cardiovascular disease or another type of major diet-related disease, there is really no need to go on a super low-fat diet. In fact, for women of childbearing age, it is important to maintain a healthy amount of fat in the diet to help support a healthy pregnancy and then to create the fat stores needed for nursing. Fats, especially the right types of fats, are incredibly important to how our bodies function. Fat in the form of fatty acids is the main energy source for the heart, which is why you've been hearing so much about essential fatty acids like omega-3s lately. These important fats are found in nuts, seeds, in some vegetables in small amounts, and even in blue-green algae. In fact, blue-green algae are the best vegan source for DHA and EPA, which support everything from heart function to brain function.

There's no magic number when it comes to how much fat should be in your diet, but a good range is anywhere from 20 to 30 percent of your calories. As a vegan who is eating a healthy, whole foods diet, you will probably come in at the lower end of this range, even if you do sneak in the occasional French fry or fried donut.

CARBOHYDRATES

"I could never be vegan—you guys eat too many carbs and if I ate that many carbs I would gain tons of weight." This is a line I have heard again and again from people who are loyal to a high-protein diet and/or convinced that carbohydrates will magically make a person gain weight. As we've already discussed, the only thing that will make you gain weight is taking in more calories than your body can burn off in a day. It doesn't matter whether those calories are from carbohydrates, fat, or protein; if you eat more of them than you need, you will gain weight.

Take me as an example: Apart from my nose dive into candy land shortly after becoming vegan, I've never been one to consistently overeat, and through all my incarnations—from omnivore while growing up, to vegetarian in my early twenties, to vegan—I have remained at a pretty stable weight. In other words, whether I was eating mostly carbs or lots of protein at any given time, my weight didn't shift dramatically in either direction, because I wasn't eating too much overall. The fact is, we need carbohydrates. They contain our bodies' primary source of fuel: glucose, or blood sugar. Our brain can't run on anything else. The only real problem with car-bohydrates is that more often than not we get our carbohy-drates refined and wrapped up in lots of fat and sugar. And this isn't exclusive to desserts. This is the case with breakfast cereals, breads, and other enriched grain products. You hardly ever hear someone say how they just gained a bunch of weight from eating brown rice and whole-grain whole wheat bread. This is mostly because we don't tend to pair these types of foods with lots of sugar and fat, but people also don't tend

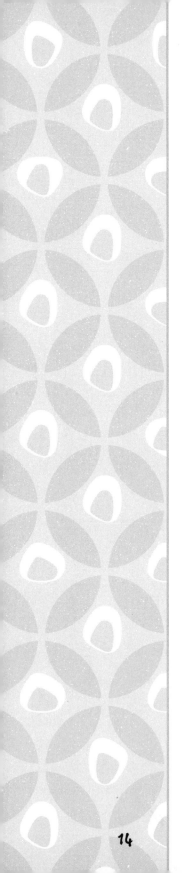

to overindulge in rich whole grains like brown rice, whole-grain whole wheat breads, quinoa, bulgur, and so on. It's not because these foods aren't delicious—they are actually super scrumptious. It's because these foods contain loads of fiber that fill you up quickly, giving you a satisfied feeling that even ten cupcakes couldn't do.

Cupcakes, cookies, and pastries have their place, too. The trick, of course, is to limit the amount of these sweet indulgences that you eat. One or two cupcakes won't really make or break your diet, but five or six cupcakes will put a serious dent in your daily caloric intake that won't leave much room for more nutrient-rich foods So, instead of beating up on carbs in general, try switching to whole-grain carbohydrates like the ones I use in this book, and leave the sweets and refined carbs as treats.

FIBER

There is a lot of buzz about fiber these days, and rightfully so. Fiber has been shown to help with digestive disorders such as constipation, diverticulosis, and hemorrhoids, as well as act as a protective agent against colon cancer. Not only that but fiber helps lower cholesterol by slowing the absorption of cholesterol and may improve blood sugar tolerance by delaying glucose absorption. Fiber is also important in weight management as it creates a feeling of fullness in the stomach and helps maintain the feeling of fullness longer. Studies have shown that typically, if you're eating a lot of high-fiber foods you are less likely to reach for foods that are laden with fats and sugars. The best part is that fiber is only found in plant foods, so by eating a plant-based diet you are well on your way to eating a fiber rich diet and reaping all the health benefits that comes with it. The Daily Recommended Intake (DRI) for fiber is 38 grams for men aged 14 to 50 and 25 grams for women aged 14 to 50.

SUGAR

Just like carbohydrates, sugar is not the enemy. Sugar is the body's source of quick energy and the brain's only source of fuel. This is why after skipping a meal, such as breakfast, you find yourself craving carbohydrates, the sugary the better. What your body is saying to you is, "I need energy now!" and your body knows that sugar is the quickest way to get every cell in your body the energy boost it needs quickly and efficiently. The USDA has not set any specific recommendations for sugar intake, they simply advise that you limit the amount of added sugars in your diet. The World Health Organization (WHO) recommends that we limit our intake of added sugars to 10 percent of our daily calorie intake. So, if you're eating a 2,000 calorie diet this allows for 200 calories from added sugars. To put this in perspective, a typical commercial soda (which is made up entirely of sugar, usually in the form of high fructose corn syrup) has about 240 calories and 65 grams of sugar. Keep in mind this guideline only pertains to *added* sugars in the diet. Naturally occurring sugars in fruits and vegetables are perfectly fine.

CALCIUM

Getting plenty of calcium in a vegan diet is much simpler than milk-drinking omnivores or cheese-loving vegetarians would have you believe. The best part is that vegan sources of calcium aren't usually connected with high-fat foods like dairy products. Fortified orange juices, fortified nondairy milks, collard greens, instant oatmeal, figs, and legumes are all excellent sources of calcium.

Calcium needs change as you age, and they vary by sex. The table on page 16 gives recommended daily allowances of calcium based on these factors. Currently, the information on food nutrition labels is based on a recommended daily allowance of 1,000 milligrams of calcium, so if a label indicates a product has "30%" calcium in it, that means a single serving provides you with about 300 milligrams. Our bodies can only absorb somewhere between 300 mg to 500 mg of calcium in one sitting, so it won't do you any good to try to guzzle down 3 cups of almond milk in a sitting to get all your calcium for the day.

When it comes to vitamin and mineral absorption, the importance of a balanced diet cannot be stressed enough. Our bodies are designed to get a little bit of a nutrient from one source, a little from another, and a little more from another. We aren't supposed to get 100 percent of the daily recommended amount of anything in one sitting. If that were the case then we would be able to survive all day off one meal and never get hungry. As you're flipping through the nutrition information that accompanies the recipes in this book, you'll notice an interesting thing—although some recipes might not have iron in them (usually the desserts), nearly every recipe contains calcium.

AGE	MALE	FEMALE	PREGNANT	LACTATING
1–3 years	700 mg	700 mg		
4–8 years	1,000 mg	1,000 mg		
9–13 years	1,300 mg	1,300 mg		
14–18 years	1,300 mg	1,300 mg	1,300 mg	1,300 mg
19–50 years	1,000 mg	1,000 mg	1,000 mg	1,000 mg
51–70 years	1,000 mg	1,200 mg		
71+ years	1,200 mg	1,200 mg		

IRON

Iron is another mineral that vegans and vegetarians tend to take a lot of flak about. However, the levels of iron-deficient anemia are exactly the same in omnivores and vegetarians in the United States. Iron-deficient anemia tends to be higher in women of child-bearing age because of loss of blood during menstruation, and therefore women of this age range have a higher recommended daily intake of iron. Pregnant women also have a high recommended intake of iron because they are supplying blood for more than one person. Fortified cereals, oatmeal, soy foods, beans, lentils, and spinach are all excellent sources of iron. You'll see in this book that the recipes that contain these ingredients tend to have 3 to 6 grams of iron in them, which for some age groups is close to the recommended daily allowance. The table on page 17 shows the recommended daily allowance for iron by age and sex.

AGE	MALE	FEMALE	PREGNANCY	LACTATION
1–3 years	7 mg	7 mg		
4–8 years	10 mg	10 mg		
9–13 years	8 mg	8 mg		
14–18 years	11 mg	15 mg	27 mg	10 mg
19–50 years	8 mg	18 mg	27 mg	9 mg
51+ years	8 mg	8mg		

VITAMIN B12

Vitamin B12 helps maintain nerve cells, is an important component in red blood cell formation, and is involved in DNA synthesis. It is also the one vitamin that is not available from a reliable source in the vegan diet. The fact that the plants we eat lack vitamin B12 is not a sign that we need to eat animal foods. Neither plants nor animals synthesize the vitamin—it is made by bacteria. This bacteria is found in the soil, and animals (including humans) once received this important vitamin by eating plants straight out of the ground. Unfortunately, due to many circumstances, this is no longer an option for humans. It is also not an option for factory farmed animals, which receive their daily recommended dose of vitamin B12 through supplements. Without this supplementation none of the factory farmed meat currently available would have B12 in it. Vegans also need to supplement their diets with B12 but this is becoming easier and easier to do. Many meat analogues like veggie burgers, vegan lunch meat slices, and vegan hot dogs have been fortified with B12. This is also the case for many nondairy milks, most cereals, and vegan yogurts. Nearly every multivitamin contains B12, and it is easily available as a stand-alone supplement in pill, liquid, chewable, injectable, and sub-lingual forms. It is important to note that a vitamin B12 deficiency can take up to five years to begin to show signs and symptoms; therefore vegans should be diligent about taking vitamin B12 in some form, whether it be from fortified foods or supplements.

SODIUM

The recommendations on sodium intake change nearly every year but with each change one thing remains constant: a

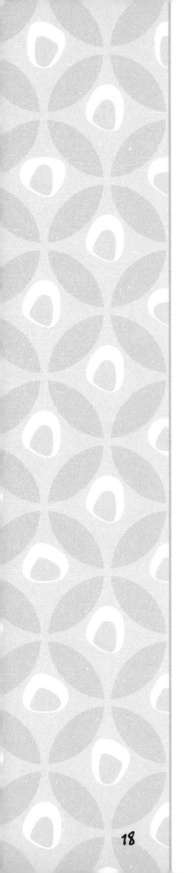

decreased recommended daily intake. Even as the recommended daily intake decreases, the actual amount of sodium a typical American consumes hovers well above 4,000 mg a day. This is nearly double the current recommendation of 2,300 mg, which is just a little less than a teaspoon of salt. For those who are 51 or older, African-Americans, and individuals with high blood pressure, diabetes or chronic kidney disease, the recommended daily intake is 1,500 mg. Making your own food is a great way to limit the amount of sodium in your diet. Over 75 percent of the sodium in the diet is added to foods by food processors—that means not only packaged foods, but also restaurant food. The best part about preparing your own food is that you have complete control over every ingredient that goes into it, including salt.

CHOLESTEROL

If you've had a chance to thumb through this book already, you may have noticed that none of the recipes have cholesterol content included in the nutrition information. There's a very good reason for that. Cholesterol is made by animals in their livers, and because plants don't have livers, plants also don't contain any cholesterol. A vegan diet is 100 percent cholesterol free, and therefore none of the foods in this book contain cholesterol.

What's That?!
A Guide to Your Vegan Pantry

Silken Tofu

Silken tofu, as the name implies, is a soft, silky version of tofu. This Japanese type of tofu adds a creamy texture to a variety of dishes like Spinach Artichoke Dip (page 103) and Fettuccine Slim-Fredo (page 158) and creates an "eggy" texture in dishes like Crustless Quiche Lorraine (page 57) and the vegan egg in Breakfast Biscuit Sandwich (page 70). Silken tofu can also be used to make soy-based ice creams, creamy dips, as an egg replacement in baked recipes, and as a good substitute for soy yogurt.

Silken tofu is available in two types of packaging: aseptic packs and 14-ounce tubs. You can usually find aseptically packed silken tofu in the same aisle as the Asian foods in your grocery store, and you can find the 14-ounce tubs in the refrigerated section near the firmer, Chinese-style tofu. The aseptically packed version has a longer shelf life and doesn't have to be refrigerated, and I like having the flexibility to use the tofu when I want to and not worry so much about the expiration date. If you choose the tub version, make sure it is *plain* silken tofu, because the tub version now comes in vanilla, chocolate, and strawberry flavors.

Tempeh

Tempeh is one of those interesting foods that some people absolutely adore upon tasting and for some it takes a while to learn to like it. Cooking preparation has a lot to do with this, and if you find yourself not loving tempeh the first couple times around try simmering it in vegetable stock before using it in a dish. This usually mellows out the bitter flavor that some report. Tempeh is made from cultured and fermented soybeans.

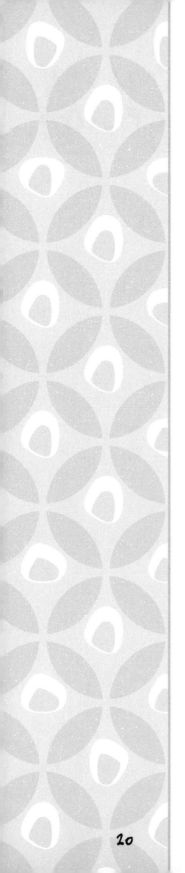

Once cultured and fermented, the soybeans are pressed into a perfect little tempeh cake ready for you to gobble up. The most commonly available tempeh in the US comes in five different varieties: soy, three-grain, flax, garden veggie, and wild rice. In this book, you can use whatever variety of tempeh you like; it will not affect the finished product.

Textured Vegetable Protein (TVP)

Textured vegetable protein (TVP) is made from defatted soy flour, and it's high in iron as well as protein. Once rehydrated, TVP takes on a texture similar to ground beef. Specific instructions for rehydrating TVP are provided in the recipes in this book that include it. For a ground-beef style, texture, and flavor to use in a recipe of your own, rehydrate 1 cup of TVP with 1 cup of dark vegetable stock and 1 tablespoon of hickory liquid smoke. This will make the equivalent of 1 pound of ground beef or turkey.

TVP can almost always be found in health food stores, either in the bulk section, in the canned beans aisle, or in the baked-goods aisle near the alternative flours. It can also often be found in conventional grocery stores, and if your local store doesn't carry it, they can usually order it for you. You can also find TVP online in various sizes and shapes.

Vital Wheat Gluten

The next time one of your friends asks you if being vegan is expensive, take a walk over to your local health food store and show your friend a bulk bin of vital wheat gluten. One pound of vital wheat gluten can cost you as little as $2 when you buy it in bulk and as little as $3 when you buy it prepackaged. Not only is it cheap, but a little goes a long way. Just ½ cup of vital wheat gluten is enough to produce a pound of Basic Seitan (page 41) or Savory Seitan (page 42). Vital wheat gluten is also extremely high in protein: ¼ cup has 23 grams. Although vital wheat gluten is used mostly to make seitan in this book, it can also be used as a binder in foods such as the meatballs in Meatball Soup (page 152).

Corn Flour

Corn flour is a whole-grain flour with a similar texture to that of all-purpose flour. It has a subtly cornmealy taste, and the light texture gives your baked goods a fluffier, less crumbly texture than cornmeal would, giving softness to recipes like Corn Flour Cupcakes with Raspberry Buttercream Frosting (page 210).

Masa Harina

Masa harina is made from corn that has been treated with a mixture of lime and water to help make important nutrients that are present in corn, like niacin, more digestible. This process also tends to make the ground end product, called masa harina, into a much finer flour than cornmeal, almost fluffy. You can immediately tell the difference when baking up dishes like Masa Cornbread (page 85). Masa is also the base of many staples of Mexican food such as corn tortillas and tamales. You can find masa harina in the ethnic foods aisle of your local grocery store with the Mexican foods.

Soy Flour

Soy flour is a high-protein flour made of ground dried soybeans. There are about 10 grams of protein in every ¼ cup of soy flour, and because it's made from soybeans it's also a good source of iron. Soy flour adds a soft, chewy texture to gluten-based sausages and seitan cutlets like Andouille Sausage (page 43) and Chorizo (page 45). Typically, soy flour can be found in the baking aisle or in bulk bins at health food stores.

Fine Sea Salt

There are so many types of salt out there—from kosher to Himalayan to iodized—it's hard to know what is what. Here's the bottom line: no one type of salt is "healthier" than the others. In every way but one, all salts are nutritionally equal. Iodized salt has the distinction of being enriched with iodine, an essential nutrient that the typical American diet doesn't include enough of. However, sea salt—and specifically fine sea salt—is my salt of choice because of its light, airy texture that dissolves quickly and evenly within a dish, creating a cohesive flavor throughout. Fine sea salt might sound ultra-pretentious, but in fact it's nothing but salt water that has evaporated to produce a wonderfully light, natural salt. I do like the security blanket of having iodine in my salt, and now we can have the best of both worlds because several varieties of iodized sea salt have become available. Although you can use any kind of salt in my recipes, I highly recommend you try out fine sea salt!

Ancho Chile Powder

Finding this smoky, mildly spicy chile powder can be difficult if you don't know where to look. The first place I recommend trying is your local international food market. They are usually filled with spices from around the world in large quantities at insanely cheap prices. If you simply can't find ground ancho chile spice in your area, you can make your own by pulsing dried ancho chiles in a food processor until they are ground to a fine powder.

Gumbo Filé

Gumbo filé is made out of the most amazing herb on Earth— sassafras. What makes it so amazing? The name of course! I'm a bit disappointed that they cover up such a wonderfully named herb with the title of "gumbo filé" but the name doesn't change its awesomeness. Gumbo filé has a spicy, earthy flavor that screams gumbo. It is also used as a thickening agent, so it should be added to dishes as the finishing touch. Gumbo filé can be found at any grocery store in the spice section.

Mace

Mace is nutmeg's older, more sophisticated sister. Both mace and nutmeg come from the nutmeg tree and are parts of the fruit of the tree: nutmeg is the inner seed and mace is the outer shell. You'll immediately be able to tell the difference between the two visually: nutmeg has a coarse appearance when ground, and mace has the texture of cinnamon and the hue of ground allspice. Incidentally, if you're ever playing around in the kitchen and want to venture out on your own with this spice, you'll find cinnamon and allspice are often great accompaniments to ground mace.

Nutritional Yeast

Nutritional yeast is an inactive dry yeast. Unlike active dry yeast, it is not alive and can no longer reproduce or ferment. What it can do is add a cheesy flavor to popcorn, soups, casseroles, salads, and steamed veggies and a creamy texture and sharp taste to staple items like Basic Seitan (page 41) and Savory Seitan (page 42). Nutritional yeast is also incredibly nutrient dense, packing in B vitamins, minerals, and 8 grams of protein for every 1½ tablespoon serving. Nutritional yeast is available in the bulk section of most health food stores. Look for the Red Star Brand, which has the highest vitamin and mineral content.

Bragg Liquid Aminos

Bragg Liquid Aminos is one of those food items that has been around for ages on the shelves of conventional and natural grocer shelves, yet I didn't hear about it until I took my first vegan cooking class back in 2006. Bragg's, as it is often called, isn't necessarily a "vegan-specific" product, but it is popular in the health food world. That's because it has the same great salty taste as soy sauce but much less sodium. Bragg's can be found in several different places at conventional and health food grocery stores. The two most popular places to find it are in the Asian foods aisle and near the salt and other seasonings.

Liquid Smoke

Liquid smoke is exactly what it sounds like: the essence of outdoor grilling in a bottle. I like to use it for the subtle umami flavors it lends to a dish, making it more savory and woodsy. I typically use hickory liquid smoke, but occasionally notes of mesquite flavors will weave their way into my cooking. When I'm making a sausage or TVP-based recipe and looking for that certain something that I can't quite put my finger on, a couple shakes of liquid smoke always solves my problem. Liquid smoke comes in four flavors—hickory, mesquite, pecan, and

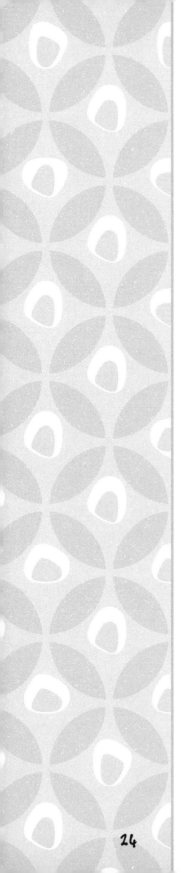

apple—but most grocers typically only carry the hickory and mesquite flavors. You can find liquid smoke in most grocery stores in the condiment aisle near the steak sauce.

Vegan Worcestershire Sauce

One of the greatest heartbreaks of my life as a vegetarian was gobbling up my favorite salad, a Caesar salad, only to be told when I was halfway through it—probably the one-hundredth Caesar salad of my life as a vegetarian—that my salad had Worcestershire sauce in it and that Worcestershire sauce contains anchovies. It never even occurred to me that the salad I loved so dearly could be secretly laced with tiny fish! As a vegan this became a non-issue since the only places I can find a vegan Caesar salad are at home and at vegan restaurants. For making my Caesar salad dressing at home I use fish-free vegan Worcestershire sauce. You can usually find it near the liquid smoke in the condiments aisle of your local health food store. Depending on the brand, the label will say either "vegetarian" or "vegan," but both brands are indeed vegan.

Vegetable Stock

Don't fret if you head to your local grocery store and can only find vegetable broth. The terms *vegetable stock* and *vegetable broth* are interchangeable. However, the type of stock or broth you use is important. I prefer to use a thin, light-colored, almost transparent vegetable stock in the majority of the recipes in this book. This type of stock adds a hint of flavor without being overpowering. A light vegetable stock is also great for cooking brown rice and quinoa instead of water to add a little extra flavor and seasoning.

I like to reserve the use of dark vegetable stock for rehydrating textured vegetable protein. Dark vegetable stock tends to have a rich, bold flavor that helps bring out the flavor in the TVP. My favorite light vegetable stock is by Swanson, and I've never met a dark vegetable stock I didn't like. The brand of dark vegetable stock available will vary by store, but most brands have a picture of the stock on the front of the package, so simply look for a deep brown stock.

Earth Balance Margarine

Replacing fats like butter in vegan recipes isn't as easy as just picking out any random tub of margarine at your local grocery store. When I became a vegan I was surprised to see that most margarines contain some type of animal product or by-product. The biggest offenders are whey and casein, which are components of milk. Earth Balance margarine is the most popular vegan margarine currently on the market. It is not only 100 percent vegan but is also relatively free of trans fats. Earth Balance can be found at nearly any grocery store or health food store. If your conventional grocery store doesn't carry it you can simply ask that they order it; it is common enough that it usually isn't a problem to order and stock. The nutrition analyses for recipes in this book using Earth Balance margarine are based on the Earth Balance margarine sticks.

Agave Nectar

Agave nectar is the hot new sweetener of the moment. Manufacturers are adding it to everything from ice cream and yogurt to bread and biscuits. However, apart from its amazing taste, there's nothing particularly special about agave nectar in terms of calories. Agave nectar is a real sugar, as opposed to an artificial or nonnutritive sweetener, and it has properties similar to many sugars with one important exception: Its glycemic index is significantly lower. Agave nectar tends to be a bit sweeter than table sugar and has a fragrantly sweet flavor. I use it not because it's the next big wonder sweetener but because of its subtle, fragrant flavor and versatility. It can be found in nearly all conventional grocery stores and health food stores in the same aisle as the sugar and other baking supplies.

Pure Maple Syrup

Maple syrup in a low-calorie cookbook—oh yes! The key to sustaining a healthy lifestyle is to make lifestyle changes that are actually doable. I personally could not live without Grade A maple syrup on my pancakes and waffles, and neither should

you. One tablespoon of pure maple syrup has only 52 calories in it, and there's a quick and easy way to make one tablespoon seem like two in the blink of an eye. I happen to have a super tiny pan that is just the thing for warming margarine or, in this case, maple syrup. If you have a tiny pan, too, simply warm the pan over medium-low to medium heat, add a tablespoon of maple syrup, then stir until thin and pour directly onto your waffles or pancakes. If you don't happen to have one of these little pans you can also warm your maple syrup in the microwave for 10 seconds at a time until it reaches the desired consistency. You'll be surprised what adding a little heat can do to stretch your syrup.

Nondairy Whipping Cream

Making homemade whipped cream is one of the most fun projects you can take on in the kitchen. All you need is the right whipping cream, a whisk and a strong arm—because it takes a whole lot of whisking to make the perfect whipped cream. As of the printing of this book there are two types of vegan whipping creams on the market: Soyatoo soy-based whipping cream and Mimic Crème Healthy Top whipping cream made of almonds and cashews. For all recipes that call for nondairy whipping cream in this book (and their accompanying nutritional information) I used Mimic Crème Healthy Top. Both it and Soyatoo are available in health food grocery stores and online at Vegan Essentials (veganessentials.com).

Unsweetened Soy Yogurt

Unsweetened soy yogurt made its way onto the shelves of health food and conventional grocery stores in 2011 and has quickly become my favorite low-calorie, high-protein alternative to vegan mayonnaise. Currently Whole Soy & Co. is the only brand in the US to make unsweetened soy yogurt, but your local supermarket can usually order it with no problem and no additional cost to you.

A Menu for Every Size and Occasion

THIS SECTION SETS you up with sample menus for four different daily calorie counts: 1,400 calories, 1,600 calories, 1,800 calories, and 2,000 calories. Four days' worth of meals are laid out for each daily caloric count, and this should be enough get you started mixing and matching recipes to create your own menus. For each recipe, the caloric count provided is for a single serving of that recipe, unless otherwise specified. Remember that when you are eating a well-balanced vegan diet, getting adequate protein should never be a problem (see page 11 for more on protein). In fact, these sample menus provide from 47 to 85 grams protein per day, with an average of 63 grams per day, which is well above the recommendations for men and women.

You don't have to follow these menus to the letter; they're simply templates to help you get started brainstorming your own daily meals. It's easy to eat healthy, low-calorie, nutrient-packed meals every day with no fuss. Not only is it easy, but you'll notice that the portions are generous, too—this will be more than enough food to keep you satisfied all day.

1,400 Calorie Menus

Day 1

BREAKFAST
355 calories / 16 g protein
> Grapefruit Brûlée (page 51)
> Naked Tofu Scramble (page 53)
> Oven Hash Browns (page 59)
> 8 ounces soy milk

SNACK
137 calories / 2 g protein
> BBQ Popcorn (page 91)

LUNCH
332 calories / 15 g protein
> Chef's Salad (page 128)
> 2 Baked Hush Puppies (page 84)

SNACK
95 calories
> 1 medium apple

DINNER
460 calories / 32 g protein
> Chili Dog (page 164)
> Cheese Fries (page 120)

TOTAL: 1, 379 calories / 65 g protein

Day 2

BREAKFAST
319 calories / 16 g protein
> Breakfast Biscuit Sandwich,
>   open-faced (page 70)
> 1 medium pear
> 8 ounces soy milk

SNACK
125 calories / 2 g protein
> Sticky Bun Popcorn (page 92)

LUNCH
200 calories / 10 g protein
> Taco Salad (page 130)

SNACK
243 calories / 7 g protein
> Simple Spiced Trail Mix (page 93)
> 1 cup fresh strawberries

DINNER
465 calories / 31 g protein
> 2 servings Chik'n-Fried Seitan (page 194)
> Broccoli Casserole (page 108)

TOTAL: 1,352 calories / 66 g protein

1,400 Calorie Menus

Day 3

BREAKFAST
380 calories / 17 g protein
 2 Hoecakes (page 64) dusted with confectioners' sugar
 Southwest Scramble (page 54)
 1 small tangerine

SNACK
150 calories / 7 g protein
 Crispy Chile Peas (page 94)

LUNCH
412 calories / 7 g protein
 Black-Eyed Pea Soup (page 149)
 Amaranth-Quinoa Salad (page 139)

SNACK
84 calories / 1 gram of protein
 1 cup blueberries

DINNER
341 calories / 16 g protein
 Chik'n Pot Pie (page 196)

TOTAL: 1,367 calories / 58 g protein

Day 4

BREAKFAST
313 calories / 18 g protein
 Crustless Quiche Lorraine (page 57)
 Oven Hash Browns (page 59)
 8 ounces calcium-fortified orange juice

SNACK
170 calories / 7 g protein
 Sweet Peas (page 95)

LUNCH
406 calories / 9 g protein
 Chipotle Butternut Squash Bisque with Squash Seeds (page 146)
 Grandma's Yeast Rolls (page 86)

SNACK
193 calories / 4 g protein
 1 medium apple
 1 tablespoon almond butter

DINNER
295 calories / 11 g protein
 Chickpea Cacciatore (page 186)
 Sesame Broccolini (page 110)

TOTAL: 1,377 calories / 49 g protein

1,600 Calorie Menus

Day 1

BREAKFAST
388 calories / 19 g protein

Sweet Potato Drop Biscuits (page 71)
South Carolina Peach Jam (page 240)
Vegetable Scramble (page 56)
1 medium fresh peach

SNACK
205 calories / 4 g protein

Guacamole (page 99)
Baked Tortilla Chips (page 98)

LUNCH
381 calories / 15 g protein

Creamy Black Bean Soup (page 151)
Sweet Potato Salad (page 135)

SNACK
197 calories / 6 g protein

Simple Spiced Trail Mix (page 93)

DINNER
411 calories / 14 g protein

Baked Risotto (page 181)
Gingered Brussels Sprouts (page 111)
Grandma's Yeast Rolls (page 86)

TOTAL: 1,582 calories / 58 g protein

Day 2

BREAKFAST
510 calories / 17 g protein

2 Lavender Pancakes (page 62) dusted
   with confectioners' sugar
Naked Tofu Scramble (page 53)
Black Bean Sausage (page 75)
8 ounces calcium-fortified orange juice

SNACK
130 calories / 2 g protein

1 cup fresh strawberries
1 cup fresh blueberries

LUNCH
393 calories / 19 grams

Meatball Soup (page 152)
Masa Cornbread (page 85)

SNACK
192 calories / 10 g protein

Spinach Artichoke Dip with Farfalle
   Chips (page 103)

DINNER
378 calories / 29 g protein

Chili Cheese Dog (page 164)
Sweet Potato Chips (page 97)

TOTAL: 1,603 calories / 77 g protein

1,600 Calorie Menus

Day 3

BREAKFAST
395 calories / 16 g protein
> Buttermilk Biscuits (page 68)
> Bread Machine Strawberry Jam (page 242)
> Southwest Scramble (page 54)
> 1 cup fresh blueberries

SNACK
216 calories / 2 gram of protein
> Mini Zucchini Loaves (page 81)
> 1 medium pear

LUNCH
472 calories / 27 g protein
> Caesar Salad with Chickpea Croutons (page 126)
> Minestrone Soup (page 143)

SNACK
137 calories / 2 g protein
> BBQ Popcorn (page 91)

DINNER
308 calories / 19 g protein
> Cincinnati Chili (page 170)
> Five-Minute Garlic Spinach (page 106)

TOTAL: 1,528 calories / 66 g protein

Day 4

BREAKFAST
396 calories / 14 g protein
> Almond Granola (page 52)
> 1 cup fresh strawberries
> 8 ounces soy milk

SNACKS
150 calories / 7 g protein
> Crispy Chile Peas (page 94)

LUNCH
350 calories / 13 g protein
> Orange Cauliflower Soup (page 145)
> Spicy Kale Slaw (page 132)

SNACKS
252 calories / 6 g protein
> Queso Dip (page 100)
> Baked Tortilla Chips (page 98)

DINNER
494 calories / 15 g protein
> Ole-Fashioned Chili Beans (page 169)
> Masa Cornbread (page 85)
> Fried Green Tomatoes (page 118)

TOTAL: 1,642 calories / 55 g protein

1,800 Calorie Menus

Day 1

BREAKFAST
479 calories / 16 g protein

    2 Oatmeal Flapjacks (page 60)
    1 tablespoon pure maple syrup
    Southwest Scramble (page 54)
    1 medium apple

SNACK
125 calories / 2 g protein

    Sticky Bun Popcorn (page 92)

LUNCH
435 calories / 15 g protein

    Refried Bean Soup (page 150)
    Masa Cornbread (page 85)

SNACK
92 calories / 2 g protein

    2 cups fresh strawberries

DINNER
484 calories / 26 g protein

    Corn Dogs (page 162)
    Cheese Fries (page 120)

DESSERT
173 calories / 4 g protein

    Butter Pecan Ice Cream (page 200)

TOTAL: 1,788 calories / 65 g protein

Day 2

BREAKFAST
445 calories / 20 g protein

    Chorizo Breakfast Quesadilla (page 77)
    8 ounces calcium-fortified orange juice

SNACK
159 calories / 6 g protein

    3 Jalapeño Poppers (page 96)

LUNCH
432 calories / 8 g protein

    Sweet Pea Soup (page 144)
    Spiced Moroccan Salad with Ancho-
       Agave Pecans (page 137)

SNACKS
62 calories / 2 g protein

    1 cup blackberries

DINNER
480 calories / 13 g protein

    Eggplant Parmesan (page 183)
    Grandma's Yeast Rolls (page 86)
    Braised Baby Bok Choy (page 107)

DESSERT
238 calories / 2 g protein

    Butter Rum Pound Cake with Glaze
       (page 219)

TOTAL: 1,816 calories / 51 g protein

1,800 Calorie Menus

Day 3

1 cup fresh strawberries
1 cup calcium-fortified orange juice

SNACK
106 calories / 2 g protein

Sweet Potato Chips (page 97)
1 cup baby carrots

LUNCH
381 calories / 18 g protein

Yellow Split Pea Soup (page 148)
Grandma's Yeast Rolls (page 86)

SNACK
137 calories / 2 g protein

BBQ Popcorn (page 91)

DINNER
524 calories / 16 g protein

Fettuccine Slim-Fredo (page 158)
Lemongrass Soda (page 225)

DESSERT
123 calories / 3 g protein

½ cup Strawberry Jam Ice Cream
(page 203)

TOTAL: 1,799 calories / 62 g protein

Day 4

BREAKFAST
522 calories / 22 g protein

2 slices Citrus French Toast with Berry
Compote (page 72)
Naked Tofu Scramble (page 53)
1 cup soy milk

SNACK
467 calories / 7 g protein

Simple Spiced Trail Mix (page 93)
Home-Brewed Ginger Ale (page 224)

LUNCH
366 calories / 9 grams

Vegetable Noodle Soup (page 142)
Grandma's Yeast Rolls (page 86)

DINNER
311 calories / 10 g protein

Indian-Spiced Chickpeas (page 187)

DESSERT
128 calories / 2 g protein

½ cup Strawberry Cheesecake Ice
Cream (page 202)

TOTAL: 1,794 calories / 50 g protein

2,000 Calorie Menus

Day 1

BREAKFAST
504 calories / 24 g protein
> 2 Griddlecakes (page 63)
> 1 tablespoon pure maple syrup
> Vegetable Scramble (page 56)
> Black Bean Sausage (page 75)

SNACK
400 calories / 13 g protein
> Almond Granola (page 52)
> 6 ounces plain soy yogurt

LUNCH
322 calories / 16 g protein
> Andouille Gumbo (page 178)

SNACK
150 calories / 7 g protein
> Crispy Chile Peas (page 94)

DINNER
319 calories / 21 g protein
> Chik'n Curry (page 190)

DESSERT
238 calories / 4 g protein
> Cherries Jubilee (page 207)

TOTAL: 1,933 calories / 85 g protein

Day 2

BREAKFAST
509 calories / 20 g protein
> 2 Banana Nut Waffles (page 65)
> 1 tablespoon pure maple syrup
> Black Bean Sausage (page 75)
> Southwest Scramble (page 54)

SNACK
384 calories / 10 g protein
> Banana Nut Bread (page 82)
> 1 cup soy milk

LUNCH
383 calories / 26 g protein
> Ballpark Hot Dog with bun (page 161)
> Creamy Coleslaw (page 131)
> Watermelon-Basil Mock Mojito (page 223)

SNACK
192 calories / 10 g protein
> Spinach Artichoke Dip with Farfalle
> Chips (page 103)

DINNER
156 calories / 8 g protein
> 3 Crispy Risotto Cakes (page 182)
> Gingered Brussels Sprouts (page 111)

DESSERT
394 calories / 12 g protein
> Strawberry Milk Shake (page 228)
> 2 cups fresh strawberries

TOTAL: 2,018 calories / 86 g protein

2,000 Calorie Menus

Day 3

BREAKFAST
526 calories / 22 g protein

    2 Blueberry Cornmeal Pancakes (page 61) dusted with confectioners' sugar
Vegetable Scramble (page 56)
8 ounces calcium-fortified orange juice

SNACK
305 calories / 12 g protein

    Chickpea Cheese (page 101)
10 whole wheat crackers

LUNCH
286 Calories / 11 g protein

    Chili Cheese Fries (page 165)

SNACK
172 calories / 4 g protein

    4 Baked Hush Puppies (page 84)

DINNER
506 calories / 14 g protein

    Kung Pao Tofu (page 188)
Lemongrass Soda (page 225)

DESSERT
220 calories / 3 g protein

    1 Ooey Gooey (page 218)

TOTAL: 2,015 calories / 66 g protein

Day 4

BREAKFAST
680 calories / 15 g protein

    2 Fluffy Flaxseed Waffles with Agave Cream (page 66)
Naked Tofu Scramble (page 53)

SNACK
201 calories / 5 g protein

    Pepita Smoothie (page 227)

LUNCH
450 calories / 12 g protein

    3 Plantain and Black Bean Tamales (page 174)

SNACK
294 calories / 7 g protein

    Sweet Peas (page 95)
Sugar-Full Pomegranate Lemonade (page 222)

DINNER
331 calories / 17 g protein

    One-Pot Jambalaya (page 180)

TOTAL: 1,956 calories / 56 g protein

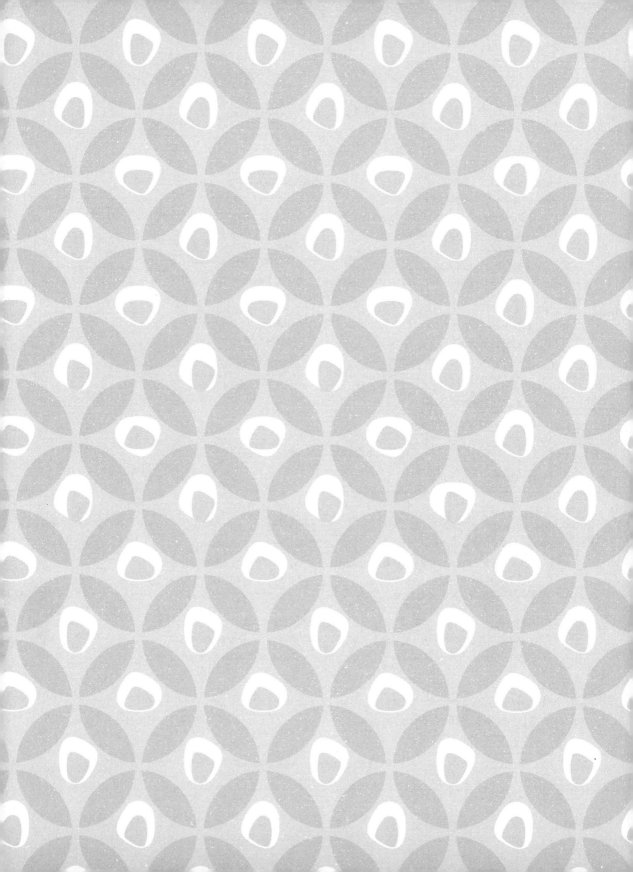

The Basics

THERE ARE TWO dishes that every vegan needs to know how to prepare: seitan and tofu. You don't need to master every variation of seitan that exists, but having a few basic recipes under your belt will go a long way towards creating flavorful, filling, low-calorie meals. Here I offer you a few of my favorite seitan and tofu preparation styles that are used throughout the book, from spicy seitan-based sausages to savory roasted tofu.

Roasted Tofu

**MAKES 14 OUNCES OR
4 SERVINGS**

I was a vegetarian for nearly four years before I found a recipe for tofu that I really liked, and I was a vegan for a full year before I began to really love tofu. The secret to beginning your love affair with tofu is to marinate it and roast it. In my opinion you can never marinate tofu long enough. I've set this marinated tofu in the fridge overnight with every intention of roasting it in the morning to throw on a Chef's Salad (page 128) for lunch, and then completely forgotten about it for the entire day! According to my taste buds, this is one of the happiest mistakes I could ever make. When it comes to roasting, however, you can definitely overdo it. Too long in the oven, and you have a dense, rubbery substance that resembles the texture of chewing gum more than a savory topping. Start checking on your tofu around 10 minutes—go ahead and pop one in your mouth to test the texture. Then you can gauge whether you'll roast for 5 more minutes or 10.

MARINADE

1 cup water

1 tablespoon plus 1 teaspoon Bragg Liquid Aminos

2 teaspoons pure maple syrup

2 teaspoons balsamic vinegar

1 teaspoon apple cider vinegar

1 teaspoon ground turmeric

1 teaspoon dried thyme

1 teaspoon dried sage

1 teaspoon dried whole rosemary

1 teaspoon dried oregano

One 14-ounce package extra-firm tofu, drained, pressed (see Cook's Tip), and cut into ½-inch cubes

PER SERVING:

113 Calories

10 g Protein

5 g Total fat

1 g Saturated fat

0 g Monounsaturated fat

6 g Carbohydrates

2 g Fiber

2 g Sugar

92 mg Calcium

2 mg Iron

322 mg Sodium

To make the marinade:

Whisk together all the marinade ingredients in a small bowl until combined.

Transfer the marinade to a shallow dish or large Ziploc bag and add the tofu. Seal the bag or, if using a shallow dish, cover with plastic wrap. Refrigerate for at least 30 minutes and up to 12 hours.

Preheat the oven to 450°F and line a baking sheet with parchment or nonstick aluminum foil.

Drain the tofu and arrange in a single layer on the prepared baking sheet. Roast for 15 to 20 minutes or until desired texture is reached.

Cook's Tip: Pressing tofu removes excess water from the tofu and allows more room for the marinade to seep into every nook and cranny and fill the tofu with flavor. In order to press tofu you can simply place it between a few clean dish towels and press out as much water as possible without crumbling the tofu.

Naked Roasted Tofu

Living meat free for over a decade has turned my relationship with tofu from contentious (to say the least) to adoring: the kind of googly-eyed love that is typically only displayed by teenagers and puppies. Although I love a good marinated tofu, like my traditional Roasted Tofu (page 38), I can also appreciate the simplicity of naked tofu, straight out the tub, slightly pressed and roasted plain. I eat it right out of the oven with just a little salt, like popcorn. And at 100 calories and 10 grams of protein a serving, it's a pretty darn good snack to munch on. If you're feeling adventurous, try this on your Chef's Salad (page 128) or even use it to top off Fettuccine Slim-Fredo (page 158) for a little textural variation.

One 14-ounce package extra-firm tofu, drained, pressed (see Cook's
Tip on page 39), and cubed

Preheat the oven to 425°F and line a baking sheet with parchment paper.

Arrange cubed tofu in a single layer on the prepared baking sheet and bake until firm, about 15 to 20 minutes.

PER SERVING:

100 Calories

10 g Protein

5 g Total fat

1 g Saturated fat

0 g Monounsaturated fat

2 g Carbohydrates

1 g Fiber

0 g Sugar

75 mg Calcium

1 mg Iron

0 mg Sodium

Basic Seitan

Everyone needs a good basic seitan recipe, and this is mine. It's incredibly versatile, easy to make, and most important, absolutely scrumptious. At only 84 calories a cutlet, this basic seitan is super low in calories, and it's off the charts in protein—19 grams per cutlet—so it makes the perfect foundation for a guilt-free low-calorie meal.

MAKES 1 POUND
OR 4 CUTLETS

SEITAN

½ cup vital wheat gluten

¼ cup soy flour

½ cup water

BROTH

2½ cups water

¼ cup nutritional yeast

2 tablespoons Bragg Liquid Aminos

1 teaspoon onion powder

1 heaping teaspoon dried sage

½ teaspoon thyme

¼ teaspoon oregano

To make the seitan:

Combine the vital wheat gluten and soy flour in a small bowl, then stir in water until it forms a ball of dough.

Knead the dough on a lightly floured surface for a little less than a minute and flatten to ½ inch thick. Cut into 4 cutlets or into desired shape (e.g. strips or nuggets). Keep in mind that the seitan will double in size during the cooking process.

To make the broth:

Combine all broth ingredients in a medium stock pot and bring to a boil. Add the seitan one piece at a time, being careful not to splash the hot broth.

Reduce the heat, cover, and simmer for 40 to 50 minutes, stirring every 10 minutes until all liquid has been absorbed. Smaller cuts like nuggets require less time, so keep an eye on them.

PER SERVING:

84 Calories

19 g Protein

1 g Total fat

0 g Saturated fat

0 g Monounsaturated fat

10 g Carbohydrates

3 g Fiber

1 g Sugar

52 mg Calcium

2 mg Iron

492 mg Sodium

Savory Seitan

MAKES 1 POUND
OR 4 CUTLETS

This may be the closest seitan gets to "beefiness." The mix of sage, tarragon, and marjoram will have your whole house smelling like a five-star restaurant. There are many ways you can use this seitan, but my favorite is to slice it thinly and use in sandwiches like Gyros with Tzatziki Sauce (page 192) and Seitan Cheesesteak (page 193).

SEITAN

½ cup vital wheat gluten

¼ cup soy flour

½ cup water

BROTH

2½ cups water

¼ cup nutritional yeast

2 tablespoons Bragg Liquid Aminos

1 teaspoon onion powder

½ teaspoon dried sage

½ teaspoon dried tarragon

½ teaspoon dried marjoram

To make the seitan:

Combine the vital wheat gluten and soy flour in a small bowl until combined, then stir in water until it forms a ball of dough.

Knead the dough on a lightly floured surface for a little less than a minute and flatten to ½ inch thick. Cut into 4 pieces then shape into cutlets.

To make the broth:

Combine all the broth ingredients in a medium stock pot and bring to a boil. Add the cutlets one at a time, being careful not to splash the hot broth.

Reduce heat, cover, and simmer for 40 to 50 minutes, stirring the broth every 10 minutes.

PER CUTLET:

83 Calories

19 g Protein

1 g Total fat

0 g Saturated fat

0 g Monounsaturated fat

10 g Carbohydrates

3 g Fiber

1 g Sugar

50 mg Calcium

2 mg Iron

492 mg Sodium

Andouille Sausage

Andouille sausage, also referred to as "hot links," is a deep, smoky, spicy, and slightly sweet sausage with French origins that is a staple of Cajun cooking. My two favorite dishes using andouille sausage are gumbo and jambalaya. Give these a try in my One-Pot Jambalaya (page 180) and Andouille Gumbo (page 178), or slice each link into thin medallions, pan-fry, stuff into a big hoagie roll, and top with your favorite condiments. You can also enjoy these as spicy breakfast sausages with a side of Vegetable Scramble (page 56). I consider these to be a mild heat, but everyone's heat threshold is different, so I recommend you test your own heat threshold by following the recipe the first time you make these. Then you can add a little more heat, if you like, by adding cayenne ½ teaspoon at a time.

1 cup vital wheat gluten

½ cup soy flour

2 tablespoons nutritional yeast

1½ teaspoons paprika

⅛ teaspoon ground black pepper

1 teaspoon red pepper flakes

¼ teaspoon ground allspice

1 teaspoon dried thyme

4 garlic cloves, minced

½ cup plus 1 tablespoon water

1 tablespoon Bragg Liquid Aminos

¼ cup ketchup

1 tablespoon extra virgin olive oil

2 tablespoons vegan Worcestershire sauce

¾ teaspoon hickory liquid smoke

Combine the vital wheat gluten, soy flour, nutritional yeast, paprika, black pepper, red pepper flakes, allspice, and thyme in a medium bowl and set aside.

Whisk together the garlic, water, liquid aminos, ketchup, olive oil, Worcestershire sauce, and liquid smoke in a small

MAKES 4 SAUSAGES

PER SAUSAGE:

222 Calories

32 g Protein

5 g Total fat

1 g Saturated fat

0 g Monounsaturated fat

18 g Carbohydrates

4 g Fiber

7 g Sugar

89 mg Calcium

4 mg Iron

619 mg Sodium

bowl. Add this wet mixture to the flour mixture and mix well, forming a dough.

Divide the dough into 4 balls, then roll each ball into a 6-inch log. Place each sausage on a separate piece of aluminum foil and wrap tightly. Twist the ends of the foil to seal. (If you don't wrap the sausages tightly enough in the foil, they will burst out during cooking).

Place the sausages into a steamer and steam for 40 minutes. Remove them from the steamer and allow to cool, still in foil. Remove foil and refrigerate until ready to eat.

Chorizo

Although the term "chorizo" has become a catch-all for the spicy, bright red sausage found in several styles of Latin cooking, not all chorizos are alike. Mexican chorizo incorporates red chile peppers while Spanish-style chorizo is rich and smoky. I can never seem to choose which one I love the most, so when I make chorizo I combine the two styles to make this bold, spicy sausage with just a hint of smoke that goes perfectly in Chorizo Breakfast Quesadilla (page 77). You can also chop up a couple of links of chorizo, pan-fry, stuff into corn tortilla shells, and top with tomatoes, lettuce, and avocado to make a delicious low-calorie, high-protein meal.

MAKES 4 SAUSAGE LINKS

1 cup vital wheat gluten

½ cup soy flour

2 tablespoons nutritional yeast

1½ teaspoons paprika

½ teaspoon red pepper flakes

¼ teaspoon ground coriander

1 to 1½ teaspoon chili powder

½ teaspoon oregano

2 garlic cloves, minced

½ cup plus 1 tablespoon water

1 tablespoon Bragg Liquid Aminos

¼ cup ketchup

1 tablespoon extra virgin olive oil

1 teaspoon vegan Worcestershire sauce

¾ teaspoon hickory liquid smoke

PER SAUSAGE:

214 Calories

32 g Protein

5 g Total fat

1 g Saturated fat

0 g Monounsaturated fat

18 g Carbohydrates

4 g Fiber

6 g Sugar

85 mg Calcium

3 mg Iron

462 mg Sodium

Combine the vital wheat gluten, soy flour, nutritional yeast, paprika, red pepper flakes, coriander, chili powder, and oregano in a medium bowl and set aside.

Whisk together the garlic, water, liquid aminos, ketchup, olive oil, Worcestershire sauce, and liquid smoke in a small bowl. Add this wet mixture to the flour mixture and mix well, forming a dough.

Divide the dough into 4 balls then roll each ball into a 6-inch log. Place each sausage on a separate piece of aluminum foil and wrap tightly. Twist the ends of the foil to seal. (If you don't wrap the sausages tightly enough in the foil, they will burst out during cooking.)

Place sausages into a steamer and steam for 40 minutes. Remove them from the steamer and allow to cool, still in foil. Remove foil and refrigerate until ready to eat.

Sweet Seitan Sausage

This seitan is inspired by Taymer Mason, author of Caribbean Vegan. *I've been playing around with a sweet seitan recipe for years, but I couldn't put my finger on the missing ingredient—until I tried Taymer's vegan ham. The secret: pineapple juice! I know it might seem like a waste of resources to buy a liter of pineapple juice just to make a couple sausages—and it totally is! Instead, look for those small 6- to 8-ounce cans or bottles of pineapple juice, then use a little to make this sausage (or use a lot by doubling the recipe). You can sip the rest or, even better, use it as a base for a sweet tropical smoothie.*

1 cup vital wheat gluten

½ cup soy flour

2 tablespoons nutritional yeast

¾ teaspoon smoked paprika

⅛ teaspoon ground allspice

1 garlic clove, minced

½ cup plus 1 tablespoon water

1 tablespoon Bragg Liquid Aminos

2 tablespoons ketchup

1 tablespoon extra virgin olive oil

2 tablespoons pineapple juice

1 tablespoon agave nectar

½ teaspoon hickory liquid smoke

Combine the vital wheat gluten, soy flour, nutritional yeast, paprika, and allspice in a medium bowl and set aside.

Whisk together the garlic, water, liquid aminos, ketchup, olive oil, pineapple juice, agave nectar, and liquid smoke in a small bowl. Add this wet mixture to the flour mixture and mix well, forming a dough.

Divide the dough into 4 balls, then roll each ball into a 6-inch log. Place each sausage on a separate piece of aluminum foil and wrap tightly. Twist the ends of the foil to seal. (If you don't wrap the sausages tightly enough in the foil they will burst out during cooking.)

MAKES 4 SAUSAGES

PER SAUSAGE:

220 Calories

31 g Protein

4 g Total fat

1 g Saturated fat

0 g Monounsaturated fat

20 g Carbohydrates

3 g Fiber

9 g Sugar

79 mg Calcium

3 mg Iron

339 mg Sodium

Place sausages into a steamer and steam for 40 minutes. Remove them from the steamer and allow to cool, still in foil. Remove foil and refrigerate until ready to eat.

Rise and Dine

LEAVING THE HOUSE without breakfast simply isn't an option. Whether you get four hours of sleep or ten, when you wake up in the morning your body is craving some food to recharge it from the long night. While you were tossing, turning, and dreaming of singing a duet with Justin Bieber, your body was busy at work. During sleep your blood pressure drops, your heart beat slows, and your muscles relax to allow your body to focus on repairing and restoring itself. And while your subconscious mind is working hard in dreamland, the rest of your brain is filing

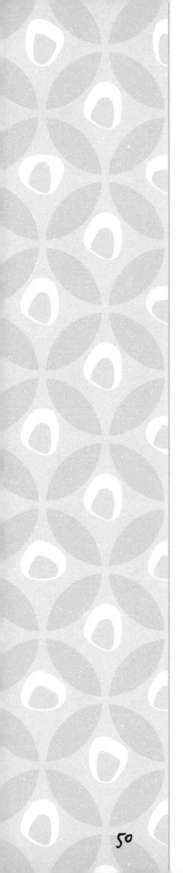

through all the things you've done in the day, deciding what to store in long-term memory and what to erase. After all this hard work, don't you think your body deserves a little more than a soy latte with a double shot of espresso for breakfast?

Studies have shown that, along with its other benefits, eating a healthy, well-balanced breakfast improves your concentration and performance throughout the day, gives you more strength and endurance for physical activity (helps you move your butt!), and even lowers your cholesterol levels. If you skip breakfast, you are very literally asking your body to make last night's dinner last all the way to lunch. No matter how filling your meal was twelve hours ago, it simply isn't going to get you through the next day. People who skip breakfast also tend to have less nutrient-dense lunches and to choose unhealthier snack options than those who eat breakfast. That's because typically, when the body has gone too long without food, the first thing it wants is simple sugars that can quickly be converted to energy. The hungrier you get, the more appealing that six-pack of Oreo cookies in the vending machine will start to look—even more appealing than the nice big Caesar Salad with Chickpea Croutons (page 126) you brought for lunch. Here are twenty-one breakfast options to get you started in the morning and help keep you full and focused throughout the day.

Grapefruit Brûlée

Looking for a way to use that blowtorch you've had sitting around the house for years? Well, have I got the recipe for you! This grapefruit brûlée's crust of torched brown sugar, mace, and allspice is a cut above your typical white-sugar version, giving the brûlée a rich caramel color and the perfect touch of Caribbean-inspired spices. If you don't happen to have a blowtorch sitting around the house, might I suggest buying yourself a culinary torch. They're only $15 to $30, and they make it easy to prepare show-stopping dishes like this one in front of friends and family. Also, culinary torches are nice and small, so they can be tucked neatly out of the reach of little hands.

2 ruby red grapefruits, chilled

1 tablespoon granulated sugar

1 tablespoon light brown sugar

⅛ teaspoon ground mace

⅛ teaspoon ground allspice

Halve each grapefruit. To loosen the segments, first cut around the perimeter just inside the skin with a paring or grapefruit knife, then run the knife along both sides of each membrane. Leave the loosened segments in place.

Combine the granulated sugar, brown sugar, mace, and all-spice in a small bowl and sprinkle each grapefruit half evenly with the sugar mixture. Using a culinary torch, melt the sugar to form a golden brown and crispy surface and serve immediately.

MAKES 4 SERVINGS

PER SERVING:

78 Calories

1 g Protein

0 g Total fat

0 g Saturated fat

0 g Monounsaturated fat

20 g Carbohydrates

2 g Fiber

18 g Sugar

23 mg Calcium

0 mg Iron

1 mg Sodium

Almond Granola

Granola has become a catch-all term for the boring things in life, yet actual granola is anything but! Granola is an amazingly versatile dish that you can eat alone, mixed with nondairy yogurt, or with your favorite nondairy milk as a cereal. It is also amazing over vegan vanilla ice cream with fresh berries. Don't be scared off by the high-calorie ingredients like almonds and dried fruits: a single serving of this granola has only 250 calories, which makes it not only a great breakfast but also a wonderfully nutritious and convenient snack for munching throughout the day.

¾ cup quick oats

2 tablespoons ground flaxseeds

2½ cups sliced almonds

½ teaspoon ground cinnamon

¼ cup dried cranberries or dried currants

¼ cup chopped sweetened dried apricots or pitted prunes

¼ cup pure maple syrup

1 tablespoon canola oil

Preheat the oven to 350°F. Lightly oil a baking sheet or line with parchment paper.

Stir together oats, flaxseeds, almonds, cinnamon, cranberries, and apricots until well combined. Stir in the maple syrup and oil until the granola mixture is completed coated.

Transfer the granola mixture to the prepared baking sheet. Bake for 10 minutes, stir, then bake for an additional 10 minutes.

Remove from the oven and allow to cool completely. Transfer to an airtight container. This granola can be stored for up to a week at room temperature.

PER SERVING:
250 Calories
7 g Protein
11 g Total fat
1 g Saturated fat
0 g Monounsaturated fat
33 g Carbohydrates
5 g Fiber
15 g Sugar
58 mg Calcium
2 mg Iron
6 mg Sodium

Naked Tofu Scramble

When I first transitioned to being vegan, I liked my tofu scramble heavily flavored with all sorts of herbs and spices. Now I also enjoy a more dressed-down version with just a hint of flavor from bell pepper and a couple of simple spices.

1 tablespoon canola oil

½ cup chopped bell pepper, any color

One 14-ounce package firm tofu, drained, pressed (see Cook's Tip on page 39), and crumbled

¼ teaspoon garlic powder

½ teaspoon onion powder

¼ teaspoon mustard powder

1 teaspoon fine sea salt

Freshly ground black pepper

Warm the canola oil in a medium saucepan over medium heat. Add the bell pepper and cook until tender, about 3 minutes. Add the crumbled tofu and cook for 1 minute, then add the garlic powder, onion powder, mustard powder, and salt. Cook, stirring often, for 5 minutes or until the desired texture is reached. Season with black pepper.

MAKES 4 SERVINGS

PER SERVING:

98 Calories

7 g Protein

6 g Total fat

1 g Saturated fat

0 g Monounsaturated fat

4 g Carbohydrates

1 g Fiber

2 g Sugar

35 mg Calcium

1 mg Iron

626 mg Sodium

Southwest Scramble

It never ceases to amaze me how many servings you can get by combining a little tofu with beans and vegetables. Get out the biggest skillet in your arsenal for this one, because it will fill up quickly. The combination of tofu, beans, tomato, and corn is so filling that I usually find myself eating just a serving of Southwest Scramble, a piece of fruit, and maybe a nibble or two of toast before I am completely stuffed. At only 136 calories and a full 12 grams of protein per serving, it's hard to beat this dish nutritionally. Just to put it in perspective, it has the same amount of protein as two large scrambled eggs but with 50 fewer calories, half the fat, and a quarter of the saturated fat. Plus, it has lots of fiber (eggs don't have any). This Southwest Scramble beats scrambled eggs hands down!

1 tablespoon canola oil

½ cup diced Spanish, white, or yellow onion

½ large red bell pepper, diced

½ Fresno or jalapeño pepper, seeded and minced

2 garlic cloves, minced

One 14-ounce package extra-firm tofu, drained, lightly pressed (see Cook's Tip on page 39), and cut into ½-inch cubes

½ teaspoon chili powder

2 teaspoons ground cumin

1 teaspoon dried oregano

1 teaspoon paprika

¾ teaspoon fine sea salt

½ cup cooked black beans

½ medium tomato, diced

½ cup cooked corn

½ cup roughly chopped cilantro

¼ cup nutritional yeast

PER SERVING:

136 Calories

12 g Protein

6 g Total fat

1 g Saturated fat

2 g Monounsaturated fat

14 g Carbohydrates

5 g Fiber

2 g Sugar

78 mg Calcium

2 mg Iron

304 mg Sodium

Heat the oil in a large skillet over medium-high heat. Add the onion, bell pepper, Fresno pepper, and garlic and cook until the vegetables have softened, about 4 to 5 minutes.

Add cubed tofu and stir to combine. Add chili powder, cumin, oregano, paprika, salt, black beans, and tomato and cook, stirring often, for 5 to 10 minutes until the tofu reaches the desired texture. Stir in corn and cook until warmed through, about 2 to 3 minutes.

Remove the scramble from the heat and stir in cilantro and nutritional yeast. Serve warm.

Vegetable Scramble

Transitioning to a vegan lifestyle and diet doesn't automatically ensure that you will eat the recommended daily minimum of five or more servings of fruits and vegetables. Vegan convenience foods are popping up on shelves all over the country, and most of them are soy or gluten based rather than vegetable based. It's important to sneak in nutrient-rich whole foods like vegetables, fruits, whole grains, and legumes throughout the day, and a Vegetable Scramble for breakfast will start you off on the right track. This scramble makes four generous, filling servings that will keep your belly full at only 169 calories a serving. You'll be smiling until lunch time.

1 tablespoon canola oil

½ cup diced Spanish, white, or yellow onion

1 small zucchini, diced

1 small summer squash, diced

1 medium carrot, peeled and shredded

1 cup diced cremini mushrooms

2 garlic cloves, minced

One 14-ounce package extra-firm tofu, drained and lightly pressed
   (see Cook's Tip on page 39)

½ teaspoon red pepper flakes

2 teaspoons ground cumin

1 teaspoon dried thyme

1 teaspoon paprika

¾ teaspoon fine sea salt

¼ cup nutritional yeast

PER SERVING:

169 Calories

16 g Protein

9 g Total fat

1 g Saturated fat

0 g Monounsaturated fat

14 g Carbohydrates

5 g Fiber

3 g Sugar

120 mg Calcium

3 mg Iron

463 mg Sodium

Warm oil in a skillet over medium-high heat. Add the onion, zucchini, squash, carrot, mushrooms, and garlic. Cook until the vegetables have softened, about 4 to 5 minutes.

Crumble the tofu into the skillet. The chunks should be small to medium so they will cook quickly. Stir to combine with the vegetables. Add the red pepper flakes, cumin, thyme, paprika, and salt and cook, stirring often, for 5 to 10 minutes until the tofu reaches the desired texture.

Remove the scramble from the heat, add the nutritional yeast, and stir thoroughly to combine. Serve warm.

Crustless Quiche Lorraine

Quiche Lorraine is one of the quintessential quiches. Look inside any of your grandmother's old cookbooks and you'll find a recipe for Quiche Lorraine. The ingredients are simply an egg custard base and bacon. Of course, neither of these items are getting anywhere near my vegan kitchen, so I've replaced the egg with silken tofu and the bacon with sweet seitan. The result is a Quiche Lorraine even your grandmother would love.

MAKES 8 SERVINGS

Two 12-ounce packages extra-firm silken tofu

1 tablespoon tahini

3 tablespoons potato starch or cornstarch

1 teaspoon fine sea salt

¼ teaspoon ground turmeric

½ teaspoon onion powder

½ cup nutritional yeast

¼ teaspoon dry mustard

¼ teaspoon original Spike all-purpose seasoning

⅛ teaspoon ground nutmeg

⅛ teaspoon ground black pepper

1 tablespoon canola oil

½ cup diced white onion

1 log Sweet Seitan Sausage (page 47), diced

2 garlic cloves, minced

Put the tofu, tahini, potato starch, salt, turmeric, onion powder, nutritional yeast, mustard, Spike seasoning, nutmeg, and black pepper into a blender and blend until smooth. Scrape the mixture into a large bowl and set aside.

Preheat the oven to 375°F. Spray a 9-inch springform pan with nonstick cooking spray.

Warm the canola oil over medium to medium-high heat in a large skillet. Add the onion and seitan and cook for 3 to 4 minutes or until the onions are translucent. Add the garlic and cook for an additional 2 to 3 minutes. Add the onion-seitan mixture to the tofu mixture and combine well.

Transfer the quiche mixture into the prepared springform

PER SERVING:

117 Calories

15 g Protein

5 g Total fat

1 g Saturated fat

2 g Monounsaturated fat

13 g Carbohydrates

3 g Fiber

1 g Sugar

48 mg Calcium

2 mg Iron

418 mg Sodium

pan and bake for 35 to 40 minutes until the filling is firm and a toothpick inserted into the center comes out clean.

Cool for 10 to 15 minutes. Remove the sides from the pan and transfer the quiche to a serving dish. Serve warm or at room temperature.

Oven Hash Browns

I highly recommend grating these potatoes with the grating blade of your food processor; it will cut your prep time in half and release a lot less water. If you don't have a food processor and have to grate the potatoes by hand, be sure to squeeze out any excess liquid before cooking. Neglecting to remove excess liquid will change the cooking time and final texture of your hash browns. Pop these into the oven before you prepare the rest of your breakfast and it'll be one less thing to watch on the stove.

¼ small white or yellow onion, grated

1 pound Yukon Gold potatoes, scrubbed and grated

½ teaspoon fine sea salt

1 tablespoon canola oil

Preheat the oven to 425°F. Line a baking sheet with nonstick foil or parchment paper and spray with nonstick cooking spray.

Put the onion, potatoes, salt, and oil in a large bowl and toss to coat. Spoon mounds of potato mixture onto the baking sheet, about ⅓ cup each and spaced apart.

Bake for 15 minutes, then turn the mounds over and press them with a spatula to flatten into rounds about an inch high. Bake until golden and crisp around edges, about 30 minutes longer.

MAKES 7 HASH BROWNS

PER HASH BROWN:

79 Calories

1 g Protein

2 g Total fat

0 g Saturated fat

0 g Monounsaturated fat

14 g Carbohydrates

1 g Fiber

1 g Sugar

4 mg Calcium

0 mg Iron

172 mg Sodium

Oatmeal Flapjacks

MAKES 9 PANCAKES

There is nothing that fits the definition of "quick and easy" better than throwing everything in a blender, pressing the on button, then pouring the batter onto a hot griddle. Honestly, these are the easiest pancakes you will ever make. Not only are they super easy to make, but cleanup takes almost no time—since you don't have to use any bowls or a spoon, just a blender and a spatula.

½ cup whole wheat pastry flour

½ cup quick oats

1 tablespoon light brown sugar

1 teaspoon baking powder

½ teaspoon baking soda

½ teaspoon fine sea salt

¾ cup plain almond milk

1 teaspoon vanilla extract

2 tablespoons canola oil

¼ cup plain soy yogurt

Warm a griddle or large skillet. Spray with nonstick cooking spray.

Put all ingredients into a blender and blend until smooth. Pour a little less than ¼ cup of batter at a time onto the hot griddle, making sure to leave room for the batter to spread. Cook until bubbles form on the top and the bottom is lightly browned. Flip and cook the other side until lightly browned, about 2 minutes per side.

PER PANCAKE:

98 Calories

2 g Protein

4 g Total fat

0 g Saturated fat

0 g Monounsaturated fat

13 g Carbohydrates

2 g Fiber

2 g Sugar

53 mg Calcium

1 mg Iron

256 mg Sodium

Blueberry Cornmeal Pancakes

Fresh is always best when it comes to blueberries, but if they simply aren't in season feel free to substitute frozen blueberries—but only on the condition that when blueberries come into season again you promise to make dozens of these pancakes using fresh berries. These pancakes are best the day you cook them because the blueberries tend to soften the pancakes as they sit in the refrigerator. However, they freeze incredibly well, and the thawed pancakes won't have the same issue. If you choose to freeze your pancakes I recommend reheating them in the oven or toaster oven at 375°F until warmed through, about 5 minutes.

MAKES 11 PANCAKES

1¼ cup cornmeal

½ cup unbleached all-purpose flour

2 tablespoons sugar

1 tablespoon baking powder

½ teaspoon fine sea salt

1¼ cups plain almond milk

2 tablespoons canola oil

¾ cup fresh or thawed blueberries

Warm a griddle or large skillet over medium heat.

Combine cornmeal, flour, sugar, baking powder, and salt in a medium bowl. Add the milk and oil and stir until smooth. Fold in the blueberries.

Spray the hot griddle with nonstick cooking spray and ladle ¼ cup of batter at a time onto the griddle, making sure to leave room for the batter to spread. Cook until bubbles form and the bottom is golden brown. Flip and cook until golden brown, 2 to 3 minutes per side.

PER PANCAKE:

115 Calories

2 g Protein

3 g Total fat

0 g Saturated fat

0 g Monounsaturated fat

21 g Carbohydrates

2 g Fiber

3 g Sugar

76 mg Calcium

1 mg Iron

241 mg Sodium

Lavender Pancakes

When I was testing the recipes for this book, the one thing that people said over and over again was how fancy these pancakes taste for such simple ingredients. That little bit of lavender creates the illusion that you've been slaving away in the kitchen all morning with a rack of exotic herbs and spices at the ready. I have the good fortune of having fragrant fresh lavender from my local farmers' market at my disposal, but if you can't find it fresh, feel free to substitute dried. If using dried lavender, start off with just 1 teaspoon at a time—its flavor tends to be more concentrated.

1¼ cup unbleached all-purpose flour

2 tablespoons light brown sugar

1 tablespoon fresh lavender flowers

¼ teaspoon fine sea salt

1 tablespoon plus 1 teaspoon baking powder

¼ cup plain soy yogurt

¼ cup unsweetened applesauce

1 cup plain almond milk

1 teaspoon vanilla extract

2 tablespoons canola oil

PER PANCAKE:

84 Calories

2 g Protein

3 g Total fat

0 g Saturated fat

0 g Monounsaturated fat

14 g Carbohydrates

0 g Fiber

3 g Sugar

104 mg Calcium

1 mg Iron

213 mg Sodium

Warm a large griddle over medium heat.

Combine the flour, sugar, lavender, salt, and baking powder in a medium bowl. While beating with an electric mixer (or a strong arm), add yogurt, applesauce, milk, vanilla, and canola oil. Beat until the batter is smooth.

Grease the griddle with nonstick cooking spray. Ladle ¼ cup of pancake batter onto the griddle at a time. The batter will spread quite a bit, so start out in small batches to test for your desired size. Cook until bubbles form on the top and the bottom is golden brown. Flip and cook the other side until golden, 1 to 2 minutes per side.

Griddlecakes

The difference between a griddlecake and a pancake is as simple as what you cook them on. Griddlecakes are cooked on a large griddle, and pancakes are cooked in—you guessed it—a pan. Working with a griddle cuts your cooking time way down. I have a big cast iron griddle that is a permanent fixture on my stove top, and it can handle 4 to 6 griddlecakes at a time, depending on how I space them out. Another bonus of cooking on cast iron is that it adds a little extra iron to your diet.

1 cup whole wheat pastry flour

1 tablespoon baking powder

¼ teaspoon fine sea salt

2 tablespoons sugar

1 cup plain almond milk

1 tablespoon canola oil

Combine the flour, baking powder, salt, and sugar in a medium bowl. Create a well in the center and add the milk and oil. Beat until smooth, then let the batter sit for 2 minutes.

While batter is sitting, warm a large griddle over medium heat. Spray the hot griddle with nonstick cooking spray and ladle ¼ cup of batter at a time onto the griddle, making sure to leave room for the batter to spread. Cook until bubbles form and the bottom is golden brown. Flip and cook until the other side is golden, about 2 minutes per side.

MAKES 8 GRIDDLECAKES

PER GRIDDLECAKE:

83 Calories

2 g Protein

2 g Total fat

0 g Saturated fat

1 g Monounsaturated fat

15 g Carbohydrates

2 g Fiber

3 g Sugar

111 mg Calcium

1 mg Iron

257 mg Sodium

Hoecakes

Hoecakes are pancakes that have gone rogue. They look like pancakes and are made like pancakes, but they lean heavily toward the savory side and can go with any meal of the day. For breakfast, just sprinkle them with a little confectioners' sugar and you're good to go. For lunch and dinner, use them to sop up the last bits of gravy from Chik'n-Fried Seitan (page 194), or even serve them topped with a little Spiced Cranberry Sauce (page 123) to add a touch of elegance to a meal.

1 cup cornmeal

2 teaspoons baking powder

½ teaspoon fine sea salt

2 tablespoons sugar

1 cup plus 2 tablespoons unsweetened plain almond milk

1 teaspoon apple cider vinegar

1 tablespoon canola oil

Warm a griddle or large skillet over medium heat.

Combine the cornmeal, baking powder, salt, and sugar in a medium bowl. Create a well in the center of the flour mixture and add milk, vinegar, and canola oil. Stir until completely smooth.

Spray the hot griddle or skillet with nonstick cooking spray and ladle ¼ cup of batter at a time onto the griddle, making sure to leave room for the batter to spread. Cook until bubbles form on the top, then flip and cook until the bottom is slightly browned, about 2 to 3 minutes per side.

PER HOECAKE:

97 Calories

2 g Protein

2 g Total fat

0 g Saturated fat

0 g Monounsaturated fat

17 g Carbohydrates

1 g Fiber

3 g Sugar

132 mg Calcium

1 mg Iron

295 mg Sodium

Banana Nut Waffles

I'm not sure exactly when carbs became the evil stepmother of the weight loss world, but I promise that you can lose weight and still eat your fill of pancakes, bread, and, most important, Banana Nut Waffles. At only 102 calories each, these waffles are waistline friendly and full of flavor. Because they are sweet and rich, with a bit of texture from the pecans, they don't need much in the way of maple syrup and require no margarine at all.

MAKES APPROXIMATELY 12 WAFFLES

¾ cup unbleached all-purpose flour

¾ cup whole wheat pastry flour

¼ teaspoon fine sea salt

2½ teaspoon baking powder

2 tablespoons granulated sugar

1 tablespoon light brown sugar

¼ cup chopped pecans

1½ cups unsweetened plain almond milk

1 teaspoon vanilla extract

1 ripe banana, pureed

Preheat waffle iron.

Combine the all-purpose flour, pastry flour, salt, baking powder, granulated sugar, brown sugar, and pecans in a medium bowl. Create a well in the center of the flour mixture and add the milk, vanilla, and banana. Stir together until combined (it's OK if there are some lumps).

Spray the waffle iron with nonstick cooking spray and ladle into it the appropriate amount of batter for your iron, about ¼ cup per waffle. Cook according to the manufacturer's directions or until the steam begins to subside.

PER WAFFLE
(USING ¼ CUP BATTER):

102 Calories

2 g Protein

2 g Total fat

0 g Saturated fat

0 g Monounsaturated fat

19 g Carbohydrates

2 g Fiber

5 g Sugar

122 mg Calcium

1 mg Iron

174 mg Sodium

Fluffy Flaxseed Waffles
with Agave Cream 📷

Flaxseed is a phenomenal ingredient because it's rich not only in heart-healthy essential fatty acids but also in fiber. The combination of flaxseed and whole wheat pastry flour makes a fiber-filled waffle that will fill you up quickly so you won't need to eat many to be satisfied. In fact, you might find that one is more than enough. Even though just one waffle provides 20 percent of your recommended daily intake of fiber, these waffles are light and airy and require only a dollop of Agave Cream to finish them off. Before you can make the Agave Cream, you'll need to chill the nondairy whipping cream and the agave nectar in a mixing bowl in your refrigerator for a half hour.

AGAVE CREAM

1 cup nondairy whipping cream

2 tablespoons agave nectar

⅛ teaspoon ground nutmeg

WAFFLES

1½ cups whole wheat pastry flour

¼ cup ground flaxseeds

2 tablespoons sugar

1 tablespoon baking powder

½ teaspoon fine sea salt

2 cups plain almond milk

¼ cup Earth Balance margarine, softened to room temperature

PER WAFFLE
(WITHOUT AGAVE CREAM):
176 Calories
4 g Protein
8 g Total fat
3 g Saturated fat
0 g Monounsaturated fat
23 g Carbohydrates
5 g Fiber
3 g Sugar
126 mg Calcium
2 mg Iron
390 mg Sodium

PER WAFFLE
(WITH AGAVE CREAM):
291 Calories
4 g Protein
15 g Total fat
8 g Saturated fat
0 g Monounsaturated fat
35 g Carbohydrates
5 g Fiber
11 g Sugar
127 mg Calcium
2 mg Iron
390 mg Sodium

To make the cream:

Chill a mixing bowl with the whipping cream and agave nectar for at least 30 minutes in your refrigerator. Add the nutmeg and beat until stiff peaks form. Cover and refrigerate until ready to use.

To make the waffles:

Preheat waffle iron.

Combine the pastry flour, flaxseeds, sugar, baking powder, and salt in a medium mixing bowl. Create a well in the center of the flour mixture and add the milk and margarine. Beat with an electric mixer at medium speed until the ingredients are completely combined.

Spray the waffle iron with nonstick cooking spray and ladle into it the appropriate amount of batter for your iron, about ⅓ cup per waffle. Cook according to manufacturer's directions or until steam begins to subside.

Top each waffle with a dollop of Agave Cream.

Buttermilk Biscuits 📷

MAKES 10 BISCUITS

Since starting my cooking blog The Lady and Seitan, which is dedicated to veganizing Paula Deen recipes, I have tried my fair share of biscuits. I promise you, I must try a new biscuit recipe every month. Of all the biscuit recipes I've made so far, this is my favorite, and although I love veganizing sweet Ms. Dean's recipes, this recipe for biscuits is 100 percent mine. Making this in a food processor will really cut your prep time, but don't let your processor run wild. If you overprocess, you will end up with a dough that is too well incorporated and wet, which will make the dough hard to work with without adding extra flour. Pulse ingredients until just incorporated, then turn the dough out onto your work surface and prep the biscuits for the oven. These biscuits are divine with South Carolina Peach Jam (page 240) or Bread Machine Strawberry Jam (page 242), but in truth, all they need is a pat of Earth Balance margarine and a side of Vegetable Scramble (page 56) to make the perfect breakfast.

1 cup unbleached all-purpose flour

1 cup whole wheat pastry flour

½ teaspoon fine sea salt

2 teaspoons baking powder

½ teaspoon baking soda

⅓ cup Earth Balance margarine

½ cup plain almond milk

¼ cup unsweetened plain soy yogurt

PER BISCUIT:

147 Calories

3 g Protein

6 g Total fat

2 g Saturated fat

0 g Monounsaturated fat

19 g Carbohydrates

2 g Fiber

0 g Sugar

77 mg Calcium

1 mg Iron

343 mg Sodium

Preheat the oven to 400°F and line a baking sheet with parchment paper.

Put the all-purpose flour, pastry flour, salt, baking powder, baking soda, and margarine into a food processor and pulse until all the margarine has been incorporated. While the food processor is still running on low slowly add the milk and yogurt.

Turn out the mixture onto a lightly floured surface and knead until the dough comes together. Flatten to ½ inch thick, then cut out biscuits with a 3-inch biscuit cutter (do not twist when pulling the cutter up). Reassemble the scraps of dough into a ball, flatten, and repeat the process.

Arrange the biscuits on the prepared baking sheet and bake for 20 minutes, or until golden and a toothpick inserted into the center of a biscuit comes out clean.

Breakfast Biscuit Sandwich

These breakfast biscuit sandwiches can be made in the traditional style with both halves of the biscuit or open-faced. If you opt for open-faced sandwiches, cut your recipe for buttermilk biscuits in half or make the whole batch and freeze the unused biscuits for another meal.

VEGAN EGG

One 12-ounce package extra-firm silken tofu

⅛ teaspoon ground turmeric

½ teaspoon fine sea salt

2 tablespoons plain soy milk

1 tablespoon nutritional yeast

¼ teaspoon onion powder

1 medium carrot, peeled and shredded

1 recipe Buttermilk Biscuits (page 68)

1 log Sweet Seitan Sausage (page 47)

To make the egg:

Preheat the oven to 350°F. Spray 10 cups of a 12-cup muffin pan with nonstick cooking spray.

Put the tofu, turmeric, salt, milk, nutritional yeast, and onion powder into a food processor or blender and blend until smooth. Fold in the carrots. Spoon the egg mixture into the prepared muffin pan. Bake for 15 minutes or until a toothpick inserted into the middle of an "egg" comes out clean.

To make the sandwiches:

Slice the biscuits in half and cut the sausage into 10 slices. Assemble the sandwiches with 1 slice of sausage and 1 egg in each.

● PER SANDWICH ●
(TRADITIONAL STYLE):

191 Calories

9 g Protein

7 g Total fat

3 g Saturated fat

0 g Monounsaturated fat

23 g Carbohydrates

3 g Fiber

1 g Sugar

100 mg Calcium

2 mg Iron

525 mg Sodium

● PER SANDWICH ●
(OPEN-FACED):

116 Calories

8 g Protein

4 g Total fat

1 g Saturated fat

0 g Monounsaturated fat

14 g Carbohydrates

2 g Fiber

1 g Sugar

62 mg Calcium

1 mg Iron

352 mg Sodium

Sweet Potato Drop Biscuits

Sweet Potato Drop Biscuits are biscuits without boundaries. Don't relegate these soft, delicate pillows to just the breakfast table. Try them as a side to Spiced Moroccan Salad with Ancho-Agave Pecans (page 137) with a tablespoon or so of Spiced Cranberry Sauce (page 123) on top. These also go well with South Carolina Peach Jam (page 240).

1⅓ cups unbleached all-purpose flour

⅔ cup cornmeal

1 tablespoon baking powder

¾ teaspoon fine sea salt

½ cup chilled Earth Balance margarine

1 cup sweet potato puree or canned sweet potato

½ cup plain almond milk

¼ cup Grade B maple syrup

Preheat the oven to 425°F and line a baking sheet with parchment paper.

Put the flour, cornmeal, baking powder, and salt into a food processor and pulse until combined. Add the margarine and pulse until the mixture resembles coarse cornmeal. Add sweet potato, milk, and syrup and pulse to combine.

Drop biscuit batter one large spoonful at a time onto the prepared baking sheet, leaving about 1½ inches of space between biscuits. Bake for 15 minutes or until a toothpick inserted into the center of a biscuit comes out clean.

MAKES 16 BISCUITS

PER BISCUIT:

139 Calories

2 g Protein

6 g Total fat

2 g Saturated fat

0 g Monounsaturated fat

20 g Carbohydrates

1 g Fiber

4 g Sugar

61 mg Calcium

1 mg Iron

275 mg Sodium

Citrus French Toast
with Berry Compote 📷

MAKES 9 SLICES OF FRENCH TOAST AND 3 CUPS COMPOTE

The calories in this recipe will vary depending on the type of bread you use. I like to make my own because this gives me complete control over the ingredients and calories. However, that's not the most feasible option for everyone so when searching for a commercial bread try to look for a bread that is not only whole wheat but whole grain. This means that, when you turn the package over and look at the ingredients, "whole-grain whole wheat" is the first ingredient. Often, a bread that advertises itself as "whole grain" contains enriched white flour, which is anything but.

The accompanying Berry Compote is also marvelous on Oatmeal Flapjacks (page 60), over Vanilla-Almond Ice Cream (page 201), or in a big bowl of steel-cut oatmeal.

BERRY COMPOTE

½ cup orange juice

¼ cup sugar

⅛ teaspoon ground cloves

⅛ teaspoon ground ginger

1 pound mixed fresh or thawed berries of any variety

1 tablespoon arrowroot powder

1 tablespoon water

FRENCH TOAST

1 cup plain almond milk

½ cup chickpea (garbanzo bean) flour

¼ teaspoon ground cinnamon

⅛ teaspoon ground nutmeg

1 tablespoon pure maple syrup

½ teaspoon vanilla extract

¾ cup orange juice

8 slices whole-grain whole wheat bread

1½ cups Berry Compote

PER SLICE
(WITH APPROXIMATELY 3 TABLESPOONS COMPOTE):

162 Calories

4 g Protein

2 g Total fat

0 g Saturated fat

0 g Monounsaturated fat

34 g Carbohydrates

3 g Fiber

18 g Sugar

36 mg Calcium

1 mg Iron

134 mg Sodium

To make the compote:

Warm a saucepan over medium heat. Add the orange juice, sugar, cloves, ginger, and berries and stir to combine. Cook until the sugar is dissolved and the mixture begins to bubble.

Whisk together the arrowroot and water in a small bowl until the arrowroot is dissolved, then whisk arrowroot mixture into the hot orange juice mixture. Cook until the sauce thickens, about 1 minute. Serve warm or at room temperature.

To make the French toast:

Whisk together the milk, chickpea flour, cinnamon, nutmeg, maple syrup, vanilla, and orange juice.

Warm a large nonstick skillet over medium to medium-high heat and spray generously with nonstick cooking spray. (Because there is no other fat in the French toast, spray the pan well and respray as necessary to prevent sticking.) Dip a slice of bread into the milk mixture and place in the hot skillet. Continue to dip and add as many slices as will fit in the pan at a time. Cook the bread until browned on both sides, about 2 minutes per side. Continue until all slices have been cooked.

Arrange French toast on serving plates and top with Berry Compote.

Chocolate Pecan Zucchini Muffins

MAKES 12 MUFFINS

I'll be the first to admit that these ride the fine line between muffin and cupcake. Let's be honest, if you put frosting on just about any muffin it would be transformed into a cupcake, and calorically speaking, most muffins and cupcakes are pretty similar. But for a little breakfast treat now and then, these muffins are perfect. The zucchini disappears into the batter as it cooks, making these muffins super moist, and they have just the right hint of sweetness and nutty goodness from the pecans.

¼ cup plain almond milk

¼ cup unsweetened applesauce

½ cup Earth Balance margarine, softened

¾ cup sugar

2 tablespoons agave nectar

2 tablespoons unsweetened cocoa powder

½ teaspoon baking soda

½ teaspoon baking powder

¼ teaspoon ground cinnamon

¼ teaspoon fine sea salt

⅛ teaspoon ground allspice

1 teaspoon vanilla extract

1¼ cup unbleached all-purpose flour

1 cup grated zucchini

¼ cup chopped pecans

PER MUFFIN:
196 Calories
2 g Protein
9 g Total fat
3 g Saturated fat
0 g Monounsaturated fat
27 g Carbohydrates
1 g Fiber
16 g Sugar
19 mg Calcium
1 mg Iron
204 mg Sodium

Preheat the oven to 325°F and line a muffin pan with paper liners.

Beat together the milk, applesauce, margarine, sugar, agave nectar, and cocoa powder with an electric mixer. Add baking soda, baking powder, cinnamon, salt, allspice, and vanilla and beat until combined. Slowly add flour and mix until just combined, then add grated zucchini and mix. Fold in the pecans with a spatula.

Divide the batter evenly among the muffin cups, filling each cup with approximately ¼ cup of batter. Bake for 25 to 28 minutes or until a toothpick inserted into the center of a muffin comes out clean. Cool completely before serving.

Black Bean Sausage

Aside from its taste, the best thing about Black Bean Sausage is its versatility. You can assemble these patties ahead of time and store them for days in the fridge, and then cook them to order every morning. Or double the batch and freeze the uncooked patties so that you always have a sausage patty at the ready. The longer these savory little patties sit in the fridge before they are cooked, the more the flavors of fennel, sage, and oregano have time to develop. You can make these up to 3 days ahead of time.

1 tablespoon plus 1 teaspoon canola oil

½ cup diced yellow or white onion

¼ cup diced green bell pepper

¼ cup quick oats

1½ cups canned or cooked black beans, rinsed and drained

1½ cups cooked brown rice

1 teaspoon whole fennel seeds

2 teaspoons dried rubbed sage

1 teaspoon dried oregano

¼ teaspoon fine sea salt

½ teaspoon garlic powder

½ teaspoon onion powder

½ teaspoon ground cumin

¼ teaspoon cayenne

MAKES 9 SAUSAGE PATTIES

PER SAUSAGE PATTY:

117 Calories

4 g Protein

3 g Total fat

0 g Saturated fat

0 g Monounsaturated fat

19 g Carbohydrates

4 g Fiber

1 g Sugar

24 mg Calcium

1 mg Iron

68 mg Sodium

Warm 1 teaspoon of the oil in a medium skillet over medium heat. Sauté the onion and bell pepper until soft and translucent, about 3 to 4 minutes. Set aside.

Pulse the oats in a food processor until they make a fine flour. Add the sautéed onion and bell pepper and the black beans and brown rice to the food processor with the oat flour and pulse until the ingredients are combined and there are no large pieces of black bean left (do not puree).

Turn out the bean mixture into a large bowl and add the fennel, sage, oregano, salt, garlic powder, onion powder, cumin, and cayenne. Combine well, using your hands if necessary. Form the sausage mixture into balls of approximately ¼ cup each, then flatten into patties. If time allows, chill patties for at least an hour or up to 3 days before cooking.

Warm the remaining tablespoon of canola oil in a large skillet or griddle (I use a big cast iron griddle) over medium heat. Add the patties and cook until brown and slightly crispy on both sides, about 2 to 3 minutes per side.

Chorizo Breakfast Quesadilla

When you plan on making these quesadillas, prepare as many components as possible ahead of time. Make your Chorizo a day or two early and have it waiting in the fridge. Make the Chickpea Cheese the night before to allow all the flavors to meld together. When it's time to make your quesadillas, all you'll have to do is wake up, take out a couple of herbs and spices, chop a little onion and garlic, and you'll be good to go.

MAKES 4 QUESADILLAS

1 link Chorizo (page 45)

1 tablespoon canola oil

⅓ cup diced yellow onion

1 garlic clove, minced

7 ounces firm tofu, drained, pressed
  (see Cook's Tip on page 39), and crumbled

¼ teaspoon ground cumin

¼ teaspoon dried oregano

⅛ teaspoon ground turmeric

⅛ teaspoon fine sea salt

¼ teaspoon red pepper flakes, optional

1 cup Chickpea Cheese (page 101)

4 large flour tortillas

Put the sausage into a food processor and process into small crumbles (about 30 seconds). Set aside.

Warm the canola oil in a large skillet or saucepan (preferably cast iron) over medium heat. Add the onion and sauté for 2 to 3 minutes until they begin to become translucent. Add the garlic and sauté for an additional 30 seconds, then add the crumbled tofu, cumin, oregano, turmeric, salt, and red pepper flakes. Cook, stirring constantly until fragrant, about 2 to 3 minutes. Add the sausage crumbles to the tofu mixture and cook for an additional minute.

Spoon ¼ cup of chickpea cheese into the center of each tortilla then spread evenly, leaving an inch around the edge.

Warm a separate large skillet over medium heat. Place 1 tortilla, cheese side up, onto the hot pan. Spoon ¼ of the

PER QUESADILLA:

328 Calories

18 g Protein

12 g Total fat

2 g Saturated fat

0 g Monounsaturated fat

39 g Carbohydrates

3 g Fiber

4 g Sugar

111 mg Calcium

3 mg Iron

611 mg Sodium

tofu-chorizo mixture onto one side of the tortilla. Fold the tortilla in half. Cook until slightly crispy on bottom, then flip and cook the other side until the other side is crispy and the cheese is melted. Repeat with the remaining tortillas and filling. Cut each quesadilla in half before serving.

Breads and Rolls

IT USED TO be that fat was the devil, then carbs took over. But when it comes down to it the recipe for weight loss, weight gain, and weight maintenance has always been the same. No matter what new fad diet rolls into town, it won't change the basic math and science. If you consume more calories than you use or burn, then you will gain weight; if you consume fewer calories than your body uses, you will lose weight; and if you consume the exact amount of calories your body needs, then you will maintain your weight. It doesn't matter if you eat a diet of pure carbohydrates,

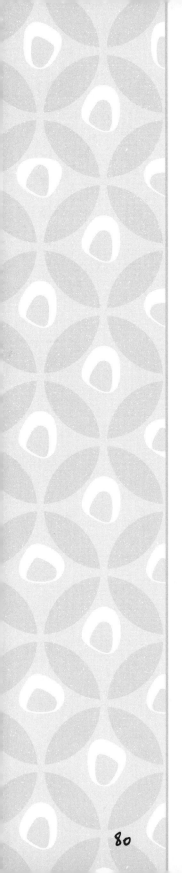

pure fat, or pure protein—when it comes to weight, all that matters is the number of calories you consume.

But it's not just about losing weight or maintaining weight—it's about being healthy, and in order to be healthy it's important to eat a balanced diet of nutrient-dense foods that have fat, protein, and—thank goodness—carbs. This means bread *is* good! Carbohydrates are the brain's principal source of energy, and without them your body has to jump through some serious hoops to get the energy it needs. So, save your body the trouble and just give it what it wants: those energizing, fulfilling, fiber-filled, B-vitamin-rich carbs!

Mini Zucchini Loaves

Fresh zucchini helps stretch this small amount of flour into 3 loaves of bread! Not only that, but when you bake zucchini into breads it has this way of just melting into the background and leaving nothing but a moist texture behind. I like to make 6, 9, or even 12 loaves of this bread in the summer when you can find huge zucchinis at local farmers' markets for super cheap. Then I freeze the loaves individually and enjoy them year-round. Each loaf makes 6 generous servings.

¼ cup canola oil

¼ cup plus 2 tablespoons unsweetened applesauce

1 tablespoon apple cider vinegar

1 teaspoon vanilla extract

½ teaspoon ground cinnamon

½ teaspoon fine sea salt

½ teaspoon baking soda

2 teaspoons baking powder

1 cup sugar

½ pound zucchini, shredded

1 cup unbleached all-purpose flour

½ cup whole wheat pastry flour

Preheat the oven to 375°F. Coat three 5¾ x 3 x 2 ⅛-inch mini loaf pans with nonstick cooking spray.

Whisk together the canola oil, applesauce, vinegar, vanilla, cinnamon, salt, baking soda, baking powder, and sugar in a large bowl until combined. Fold in the shredded zucchini, then add the all-purpose flour and pastry flour ½ cup at a time, stirring to combine between additions.

Divide the batter among the prepared loaf pans and bake for 35 to 45 minutes until the loaves are golden brown and a toothpick inserted into the center of a loaf comes out clean.

Allow to cool in the pan for about 10 minutes then run a knife around the edge of each pan and remove the loaves. Allow to cool completely before slicing and serving.

MAKES 3 LOAVES OR 18 SERVINGS

PER SERVING:
113 Calories
1 g Protein
3 g Total fat
0 g Saturated fat
2 g Monounsaturated fat
20 g Carbohydrates
1 g Fiber
12 g Sugar
36 mg Calcium
1 mg Iron
156 mg Sodium

Banana Nut Bread 📷

MAKES 12 SERVINGS

When it comes to making low-calorie food, I don't like to cut out the stuff that makes food so appealing. Fat, sugar, and flour are the trifecta of taste-bud happiness! It's all about eating them in moderation and finding lower calorie treats that are still satisfying. You don't have to be afraid of shortening, margarine, and flour, but you will get into trouble with these foods when they stop becoming an occasional treat and start to become a normal part of your diet at nearly every meal, every day. When you can, it's always a good idea to cut all-purpose flour with a little whole wheat pastry flour, which naturally has more fiber and B vitamins.

This bread freezes really well. Make a loaf, slice it up, divide it into 12 servings, and take them out one at a time to nibble for weeks to come. When reheating this bread I highly recommend defrosting and warming it in a toaster or countertop convection oven. Its buttery flavor will really come out, and you'll find you don't need anything to accompany it but a napkin and a smile.

¼ cup Earth Balance margarine, softened

¼ cup vegetable shortening

1 cup sugar

3 bananas, mashed

1 cup unbleached all-purpose flour

1 cup whole wheat pastry flour

1 teaspoon fine sea salt

2 teaspoons baking powder

½ teaspoon baking soda

½ cup plain soy yogurt

⅓ cup plain almond milk

½ cup chopped pecans

PER SERVING:

284 Calories

3 g Protein

12 g Total fat

3 g Saturated fat

0 g Monounsaturated fat

43 g Carbohydrates

3 g Fiber

22 g Sugar

77 mg Calcium

1 mg Iron

372 mg Sodium

Preheat the oven to 350°F. Spray a 9 x 5 x 3-inch loaf pan with nonstick cooking spray.

Cream margarine, shortening, and sugar together with an electric mixer. Add bananas and beat until well incorporated. One at a time, add the all-purpose flour, pastry flour, salt, baking powder, baking soda, yogurt, milk, and pecans, incorporating each ingredient fully before adding the next.

Pour the batter into the prepared loaf pan and bake for 40 to 45 minutes or until a toothpick inserted into the center comes out clean.

Baked Hush Puppies

MAKES 18 HUSH PUPPIES

As a child I had a love of hush puppies that bordered on obsession. It didn't matter how much grease was seeping through the paper tray they were served on, or the fact that one person probably shouldn't eat a dozen of them in a sitting, I just had to have them. This strategy worked fine for me as a kid, but at thirty years old, sitting down to a plateful of grease-drenched hush puppies means one thing—I won't be fitting into my favorite pair of jeans for much longer. These baked hush puppies are the answer to my prayers. Instead of dousing the puppies in oil, I just add a couple tablespoons to the batter and bake them up. They come out crispy on the outside and soft and warm on the inside, just like their fried counterparts—and you won't have to do the wiggle dance to get into your jeans tomorrow.

½ cup cornmeal

½ cup unbleached all-purpose flour

2 teaspoons baking powder

1 teaspoon sugar

½ teaspoon fine sea salt

¼ cup plus 2 tablespoons unsweetened plain almond milk

1 tablespoon apple cider vinegar

2 tablespoons canola oil

1 scallion, chopped

PER HUSH PUPPY:

43 Calories

1 g Protein

2 g Total fat

0 g Saturated fat

0 g Monounsaturated fat

6 g Carbohydrates

0 g Fiber

0 g Sugar

41 mg Calcium

0 mg Iron

124 mg Sodium

Preheat the oven to 425°F. Spray an 18-cup mini-muffin pan with nonstick cooking spray.

Combine the cornmeal, flour, baking powder, sugar, and salt in a medium bowl. Create a well in the center of the flour mixture and add the milk, vinegar, oil, and scallion. Stir until thoroughly combined. Spoon 1 tablespoon of batter into each cup of the prepared muffin pan. Bake for 10 to 15 minutes or until golden and crispy.

Masa Cornbread

All you fans of traditional southern cornbread, it's time to turn everything you know about cornbread on its head. Masa harina is a staple in my kitchen for making homemade corn tortillas and tamales. When you open up the package, masa harina will look almost identical to cornmeal, but when you rub it between your fingers you'll notice right away that masa harina is a lot softer and less grainy. The texture of the masa makes this cornbread melt in your mouth. Usually I slather my cornbread with margarine, but this bread is buttery, soft, and delicious right out the oven all on its own.

White cornmeal is gaining popularity in US grocery stores, but if you search high and low and absolutely can't find it, use yellow cornmeal instead.

1 cup masa harina

1⅓ cup white cornmeal

¼ cup unbleached all-purpose flour

3 tablespoons plus 1 teaspoon baking powder

¼ cup plus 2 tablespoons sugar

1 teaspoon fine sea salt

2½ cups plain almond milk

¼ cup unsweetened applesauce

¼ cup canola oil

2 tablespoons white vinegar

Preheat the oven to 400°F. Spray a 2-quart casserole dish with nonstick cooking spray.

Combine masa harina, cornmeal, flour, baking powder, sugar, and salt in a medium bowl. Create a well in the center of the masa mixture and add the milk, applesauce, canola oil, and vinegar. Stir until completely combined. Transfer the batter to the prepared baking dish and bake for 20 to 25 minutes until a toothpick inserted into the center comes out clean. Allow to cool in the pan.

MAKES 12 SERVINGS

PER SERVING:

162 Calories

2 g Protein

5 g Total fat

0 g Saturated fat

0 g Monounsaturated fat

28 g Carbohydrates

2 g Fiber

7 g Sugar

240 mg Calcium

2 mg Iron

603 mg Sodium

Grandma's Yeast Rolls

MAKES 12 ROLLS

I'm going to be honest with you, neither my grandma nor my Nana ever made these rolls. In fact, my grandma doesn't even let me call her Grandma—she will only answer to Grandmother. (I know it seems like a small distinction, but trust me, it's a BIG deal.) Although these yeast rolls aren't an old family recipe passed down through the generations, what better time than the present to start my own tradition by creating rolls that I can pass on to my own grandchildren decades from now?

> 3½ cups unbleached all-purpose flour
>
> 3 tablespoons sugar
>
> ½ teaspoon fine sea salt
>
> 2¼ teaspoons active dry yeast
>
> 1 cup plus 2 tablespoons water, warm if not using a bread machine
>
> 2 tablespoons canola oil

To make in a bread machine:

Put all the ingredients into a bread machine according to the manufacturer's directions, making sure the yeast is at the very top and is not touching the liquids. Start the dough cycle and allow it to go through its first rise. After the first rise is over, remove the dough. Pinch off chunks of dough and roll into 2-inch balls.

Line a baking sheet or pan with parchment paper and arrange the balls of dough in the pan. Cover the dough with a damp, light cloth or paper towel. Set the dough in a warm location and let stand until doubled in size, about 40 to 45 minutes.

Preheat the oven to 325°F. Bake for 30 to 45 minutes until golden brown. Remove from the oven and allow the rolls to cool for 5 minutes before removing from the pan.

To make by hand:

Combine 2¾ cups of the flour, 2 tablespoons of the sugar, and the salt. In a separate bowl, combine the yeast and the remaining 1 tablespoon sugar with the warm water. Let sit for 5 to 10 minutes.

PER ROLL:
167 Calories
4 g Protein
3 g Total fat
0 g Saturated fat
0 g Monounsaturated fat
31 g Carbohydrates
1 g Fiber
3 g Sugar
6 mg Calcium
2 mg Iron
100 mg Sodium

Add yeast mixture and oil to the flour mixture and stir until completely combined, using your hands if necessary. Turn the dough out onto a lightly floured surface and knead, adding ½ to ¾ cup of the remaining flour as needed to prevent sticking. Continue to knead the dough until smooth and elastic to the touch, about 15 minutes. Place in a large greased bowl, cover with a dry towel, and let stand in a warm place until doubled in size, about 1 hour. Punch down the dough. Pinch off chunks of dough and roll into 2-inch balls.

Line a baking sheet or pan with parchment paper and arrange the balls of dough in the pan. Cover the dough with a damp, light cloth or paper towel. Set the dough in a warm location and let it stand until doubled in size, about 40 to 45 minutes.

Preheat the oven to 325°F. Bake for 30 to 45 minutes until golden brown. Remove from the oven and allow the rolls to cool for 5 minutes before removing from the pan.

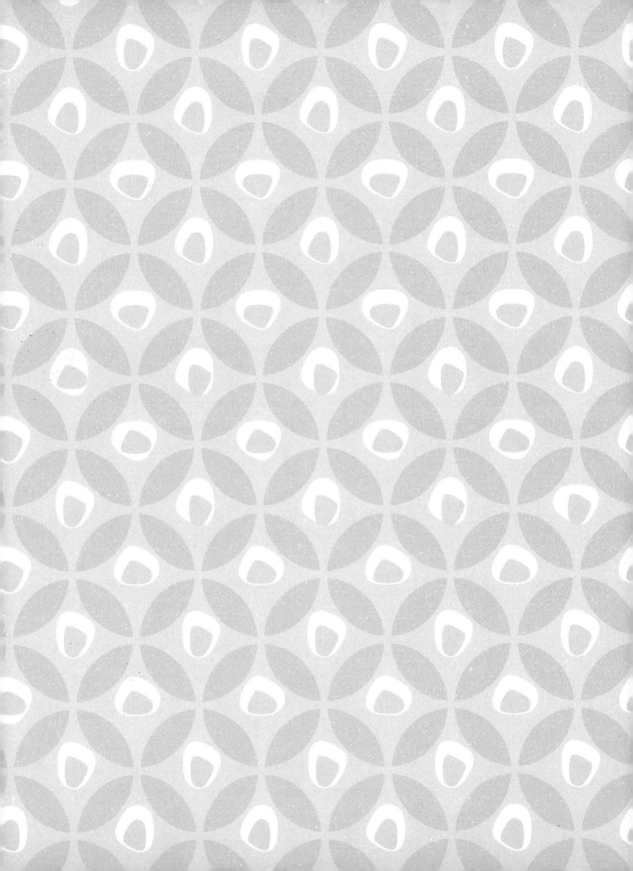

Snacks and Small Bites

ONE OF THE worst things you can do to sabotage your own weight-loss success is to skip meals or allow yourself to get too hungry. We've all been there—you had every intention of eating lunch at noon—a healthy salad, maybe a little wrap on the side, and a big bottle of water. Then someone at work calls you with an urgent request that has to be done now, or you decide to run a couple errands during lunch that take way too long and now you have only five minutes left before you need to get back to work or school or pick up the kids. By the time you finally sit down to eat over an hour later,

all you want is something deep fried and dipped in sugar, and a side of sugar with a straw in it. Every healthy intention goes out the door when your body is craving what it needs to survive, which is energy. The quickest way to get energy is through foods that have readily accessible sugars that can be easily broken down to fuel your brain and body. Sugar cravings are a biological response to hunger that you simply can't help. To avoid getting to that point, you simply have to carry snacks on you at all times. Healthy snacking is important, it keeps your blood sugar stable throughout the day so you will avoid those big dips that send you running to the vending machine.

BBQ Popcorn 📷

Here is the trick to this popcorn. You have to restrain yourself. Everyone who has tested this recipe, myself included, broke the first cardinal rule of healthy eating—portion control. I can't tell you how many times I have sat down with an entire bowl of BBQ Popcorn, started munching, and before I knew it the entire bowl was gone! At 137 calories a serving this popcorn is a wonderful snack, but if you sit down and eat the whole bowl it's nearly two meals' worth of calories! After you make this popcorn, divide it up into 8 servings in little baggies and set them aside. Keep one at your desk, keep one in your purse or man-bag, and snack on it between meals to keep hunger at bay.

⅔ cups popping corn

2 tablespoons canola oil

2 tablespoons Spanish paprika

½ teaspoon smoked paprika

¾ teaspoon fine sea salt

3 tablespoons sugar

2 teaspoons onion powder

2 tablespoons Earth Balance margarine, melted

Add the popping corn and canola oil to a popcorn machine and pop according to manufacturer's directions. Transfer to a large bowl.

Combine both types of paprika, the salt, sugar, and onion powder in a small bowl. Drizzle the melted margarine over the popcorn and toss, then sprinkle with the spice mixture and toss again to coat.

PER SERVING:

137 Calories

2 g Protein

7 g Total fat

1 g Saturated fat

0 g Monounsaturated fat

17 g Carbohydrates

3 g Fiber

5 g Sugar

6 mg Calcium

1 mg Iron

252 mg Sodium

Sticky Bun Popcorn

MAKES 4 QUARTS OR 8 SERVINGS

Sticky Bun Popcorn has all the taste of an ooey-gooey sticky bun but without the syrupy sugar and cinnamon slathered over all your fingers and half your face. If you're like me and get a sweet tooth midday, then this is the perfect snack for you. It will satisfy that sweet tooth without going overboard on the calories.

⅔ cups popping corn

2 tablespoons canola oil

¼ teaspoon fine sea salt

2 tablespoons light brown sugar

1 teaspoon ground cinnamon

2 tablespoons Earth Balance margarine, melted

Add the popping corn and canola oil to a popcorn machine and pop according to manufacturer's directions. Transfer to a large bowl.

Combine the salt, sugar, and cinnamon in a small bowl. Drizzle the melted margarine over the popcorn and toss, then sprinkle with sugar mixture and toss again to coat.

PER SERVING:

125 Calories

2 g Protein

7 g Total fat

1 g Saturated fat

0 g Monounsaturated fat

15 g Carbohydrates

2 g Fiber

4 g Sugar

6 mg Calcium

1 mg Iron

105 mg Sodium

Simple Spiced Trail Mix

It might seem counterintuitive to eat a trail mix made almost completely of fatty nuts and seeds, but there is a method to my madness. Fat is an essential element in the diet, and the healthy fats found in nuts and seeds are priceless to heart health. Besides, nuts pack a whole lot of nutritional goodness in a little package. They're full of protein, fiber, and essential fatty acids and minerals. In each serving of this trail mix (about ⅓ cup) you get 6 grams of protein along with calcium, iron, zinc, magnesium, folate, potassium, selenium, and niacin. See? Nuts aren't such a crazy idea after all.

MAKES 8 SERVINGS

¾ cup whole almonds

½ cup pecan halves

½ cup walnut halves

½ cup raw sunflower seeds

1 teaspoon canola oil

¼ teaspoon fine sea salt

¼ teaspoon chili powder

¼ teaspoon dried oregano

½ teaspoon ground cumin

Preheat the oven to 350°F and line a baking sheet with parchment paper or nonstick aluminum foil.

Combine all the ingredients in a large bowl and stir until the nuts are coated. Transfer to the prepared baking sheet and bake until fragrant, about 10 minutes. Let cool and store in an airtight container for up to 7 days.

PER SERVING:

197 Calories

6 g Protein

18 g Total fat

1 g Saturated fat

9 g Monounsaturated fat

5 g Carbohydrates

3 g Fiber

1 g Sugar

44 mg Calcium

1 mg Iron

79 mg Sodium

Crispy Chile Peas

MAKES 6 SERVINGS

I'm constantly counseling clients on the importance of incorporating beans and legumes into their diets because they are so high in protein, essential vitamins, and fiber. But sometimes even I forget what powerhouses of nutrition they are for so few calories. I make these Crispy Chile Peas at least once a week. I portion them out into baggies, store them on the countertop or in the fridge, and take them with me everywhere I go. With nearly 20 percent of my recommended daily allowance of iron, almost 25 percent of my daily recommended amount of fiber, and 7 grams of protein, this convenient 150-calorie snack is a nutrient-rich wonder.

3 cups cooked chickpeas

2 teaspoons ancho chile powder

2 teaspoons dried oregano

¾ teaspoon ground allspice

¼ teaspoon ground cloves

½ teaspoon garlic powder

½ teaspoon fine sea salt

2 teaspoons extra virgin olive oil

Preheat the oven to 400°F and line a baking sheet with nonstick foil or parchment paper.

Combine all the ingredients in a medium bowl and toss to coat. Spread in a single layer over the prepared baking sheet and bake for 25 to 30 minutes until lightly browned and crispy. Store in an airtight container for up to 2 weeks.

PER SERVING:

150 Calories

7 g Protein

4 g Total fat

0 g Saturated fat

2 g Monounsaturated fat

23 g Carbohydrates

6 g Fiber

4 g Sugar

48 mg Calcium

3 mg Iron

203 mg Sodium

Sweet Peas

I'm guilty of sitting down to late-night talk shows on my DVR with a handful of Sweet Peas and snacking on and off until it's time to go to bed. It's amazing how just 3 tablespoons of brown sugar and a little bit of Chinese five-spice can make you feel like you're indulging in a decadent treat when in fact you're filling yourself with a sincerely nutritious snack with less than 200 calories.

3 cups cooked chickpeas

3 tablespoons light brown sugar

1 teaspoon Chinese five-spice powder

½ teaspoon fine sea salt

1½ teaspoons extra virgin olive oil

Preheat the oven to 400°F and line a baking sheet with nonstick foil or parchment paper.

Combine all the ingredients in a medium bowl and toss to coat. Spread in a single layer on prepared baking sheet and bake for 25 to 30 minutes until lightly browned and crispy. Store in an airtight container for up to 2 weeks.

PER SERVING:

170 Calories

7 g Protein

3 g Total fat

0 g Saturated fat

0 g Monounsaturated fat

29 g Carbohydrates

6 g Fiber

11 g Sugar

46 mg Calcium

3 mg Iron

205 mg Sodium

Jalapeño Poppers

MAKES 24 POPPERS

I'll be the first to admit to you, there's a very long list of foods that I never tried when I was an omnivore, and jalapeño poppers is one of them. I have no clue what the cheese-laden, deep-fried version tastes like, but what I do know is that this version absolutely rocks. It's creamy, a wee bit spicy, and nice and crispy, thanks to the panko bread crumbs. Panko bread crumbs are Japanese-style bread crumbs that give the perfect texture to oven-fried foods, and you can find them in the Asian food aisle of most conventional grocery stores and health food stores.

8 ounces vegan cream cheese, softened

¼ cup nutritional yeast

1 teaspoon chile powder

½ cup plain soy yogurt

1 cup panko bread crumbs

½ cup unbleached all-purpose flour

½ teaspoon ancho chile powder

½ teaspoon dried oregano

½ teaspoon dried thyme

½ teaspoon fine sea salt

12 large jalapeños, halved lengthwise, membranes and seeds discarded

PER JALAPEÑO POPPER:

53 Calories

2 g Protein

2 g Total fat

1 g Saturated fat

0 g Monounsaturated fat

7 g Carbohydrates

1 g Fiber

1 g Sugar

21 mg Calcium

1 mg Iron

122 mg Sodium

Preheat the oven to 350°F and line a baking sheet with nonstick foil or parchment paper.

Stir the cream cheese, nutritional yeast, and ½ teaspoon of the chile powder until thoroughly combined. In a separate small bowl, whisk together the yogurt and the remaining ½ teaspoon chile powder. In a shallow dish combine the bread crumbs, flour, ancho chile powder, oregano, thyme, and salt.

Spoon 1 rounded tablespoon of the cream cheese mixture into each jalapeño half. Dip each half into the yogurt and then press into the bread crumbs to coat. Lay each jalapeño, cut side up, on the prepared baking sheet.

Bake until crispy and golden, about 30 minutes.

Sweet Potato Chips

You don't need a mandoline or a food processor with a slicing blade to slice these chips, but it will make your life much easier if you use one, and it will ensure that your cooked chips are evenly crisp.

1 medium garnet sweet potato, about ¾ pound

¼ teaspoon ground allspice

½ teaspoon ground cumin

1 teaspoon sugar

½ teaspoon chili powder

¼ teaspoon fine sea salt

Preheat the oven to 400°F. Line two baking sheets with non-stick aluminum foil or parchment paper and spray lightly with nonstick cooking spray.

Thinly slice the sweet potato and arrange in a single layer on the prepared baking sheets. Spray with cooking spray and bake for 8 to 10 minutes until the slices darken slightly.

While potato slices are baking, combine the allspice, cumin, sugar, chili powder, and salt in a small bowl and set aside.

Flip the chips over and bake until browned, about 10 minutes more. Transfer to a large bowl and toss with spice mixture.

MAKES 4 SERVINGS

PER SERVING:

71 Calories

1 g Protein

0 g Total fat

0 g Saturated fat

0 g Monounsaturated fat

16 g Carbohydrates

2 g Fiber

6 g Sugar

27 mg Calcium

1 mg Iron

174 mg Sodium

Baked Tortilla Chips

MAKES 6 SERVINGS

Making your own tortilla chips is one of the simplest things you will ever do in the kitchen, and yet anyone you serve them to will think you slaved away in the kitchen all day. For a classic combination, serve these crisp chips with Guacamole (page 99) or store-bought salsa.

12-ounce package white or yellow corn tortillas
1 tablespoon Taco Seasoning Mix (page 234)

Preheat the oven to 350°F and line a large baking sheet with parchment paper.

Cut the tortillas into wedges and arrange them on the prepared baking sheet in a single layer, overlapping a little if necessary. Spray with nonstick cooking spray and sprinkle with the taco seasoning.

Bake for about 7 minutes, then remove the baking sheet from the oven and toss the chips. Return to the oven and bake for an additional 8 minutes or until the chips are crisp.

PER SERVING:
126 Calories
3 g Protein
1 g Total fat
0 g Saturated fat
0 g Monounsaturated fat
27 g Carbohydrates
3 g Fiber
0 g Sugar
99 mg Calcium
1 mg Iron
103 mg Sodium

Guacamole

Guacamole is another classic example of the importance of portion control. Sure, most of us could eat an entire avocado in one sitting, but that's really not a proper serving. If you don't have plans to share this guacamole with three of your closest friends, I suggest dividing it into 4 portions right away. You can eat the first portion with Baked Tortilla Chips (page 98) and nibble on the remaining 3 servings over the next three days.

MAKES 4 SERVINGS

1 avocado, diced

½ fresh serrano chile pepper, seeds discarded and flesh minced

¼ cup diced white onion

2 tablespoons chopped fresh cilantro

1 whole sun-dried tomato, roughly chopped

¼ teaspoon fine sea salt

½ teaspoon lime juice

Put the avocado in a small bowl. Depending on the texture you prefer, either mash the avocado or leave it as is.

Add the chile, onion, cilantro, tomato, salt, and lime juice and mix together. Let chill in the refrigerator for 30 minutes before serving to allow the flavors to combine.

PER SERVING:

79 Calories

1 g Protein

7 g Total fat

1 g Saturated fat

0 g Monounsaturated fat

5 g Carbohydrates

3 g Fiber

1 g Sugar

9 mg Calcium

0 mg Iron

154 mg Sodium

Queso Dip

There is a very real possibility that I have lived under a rock my whole life, because I only recently realized that people will sit down to a big bowl of melted cheese and just start dipping and eating. In my world, if there are chips and melted cheese around (the vegan variety, of course), then there are nachos to be made! However, all my friends have insisted that they want a hot bowl of melty gooeyness to dip their chips in, and so, being the great friend I am, I have obliged them and created this Queso Dip recipe. Enjoy!

1 medium Yukon Gold potato, peeled and diced

1 medium parsnip, peeled and diced

½ cup diced white onion

1 garlic clove, chopped

1 cup water

½ cup cooked navy beans

2 tablespoons canola oil

¾ teaspoon fine sea salt

1½ teaspoons fresh lemon juice

½ cup cashews

PER SERVING:

126 Calories

3 g Protein

7 g Total fat

0 g Saturated fat

0 g Monounsaturated fat

15 g Carbohydrates

2 g Fiber

1 g Sugar

23 mg Calcium

1 mg Iron

272 mg Sodium

Combine the potato, parsnip, onion, garlic, and water in a small saucepan and set over medium heat. Bring to a boil, lower the heat, and simmer, covered, for 10 minutes or until the vegetables are tender.

Put the navy beans, oil, salt, lemon juice, cashews, and the cooked vegetables with their cooking water into a blender and blend until completely smooth. Transfer to a small crockpot set on low or to a fondue pot to keep warm.

Chickpea Cheese

The Ultimate Uncheese Cookbook *by Jo Stepaniak was one of my first go-to books as a new vegan trying to figure out the world of vegan cheeses. As any vegan can tell you, there is a lot of trial and error involved in finding the flavor and texture that you like. With its smooth texture and slightly sharp taste, Chickpea Cheese is the one for me. This recipe started with Jo's idea of using chickpeas as a base for cheese spreads, and over the years it has morphed into the recipe you see before you, a low-cal, high-protein dip or spread that I hope you'll love as much as I do. Try it in Chorizo Breakfast Quesadillas (page 77) or simply spread on crackers as a snack.*

MAKES 1¾ CUPS OR SEVEN SERVINGS

2 cups cooked chickpeas

¼ cup nutritional yeast

1 tablespoon white wine vinegar

1 tablespoon tahini

1 tablespoon flax oil or extra virgin olive oil

3 tablespoons water

1 teaspoon fine sea salt

1 teaspoon onion powder

½ teaspoon paprika

¼ teaspoon garlic powder

⅛ teaspoon dry mustard

Put all ingredients into a food processor and process until smooth. Store, tightly covered, for up to 1 week in the refrigerator.

PER SERVING
(¼ CUP):

109 Calories

7 g Protein

5 g Total fat

1 g Saturated fat

0 g Monounsaturated fat

16 g Carbohydrates

5 g Fiber

3 g Sugar

37 mg Calcium

2 mg Iron

344 mg Sodium

White Bean Spread

**MAKES 2 CUPS OR
4 SERVINGS**

If you couldn't already tell by thumbing through the table of contents, I'll confess, I love chickpeas. They're fantastic stirred into hearty Chickpea Cacciatore (page 186) and roasted for Crispy Chile Peas (page 94), but I decided my love for chickpeas needed some limits when I looked into my fridge and saw five different chickpea dishes. I decided enough was enough and it was time to show a little love to the other legumes in my life, like the time-honored navy bean. Navy beans are extremely versatile and a great base layer for other flavors, whether in Backyard Beans (page 167) or in this smooth, subtle spread.

1½ cups cooked navy beans

3 tablespoons nutritional yeast

1 tablespoon tahini

2 teaspoons white wine vinegar

1½ teaspoons white miso

¾ teaspoon onion powder

¼ teaspoon fine sea salt

¼ teaspoon paprika

¼ teaspoon garlic powder

¼ teaspoon dry mustard

2 tablespoons flax oil

Put all the ingredients into a food processor and process until smooth. Store, tightly covered, for up to 1 week in the refrigerator.

PER SERVING
(½ CUP):
125 Calories
10 g Protein
3 g Total fat
0 g Saturated fat
1 g Monounsaturated fat
23 g Carbohydrates
6 g Fiber
0 g Sugar
71 mg Calcium
2 mg Iron
233 mg Sodium

Spinach Artichoke Dip
with Farfalle Chips

Anything would taste good deep fried and then plunged into a creamy, fat-based dip, but what happens when you take away all the cream, butter, and cheese that traditional spinach artichoke dip is based on and nix the deep-fried tortilla chips it is usually served with? Can it possibly be good? You bet! I've replaced the traditional tortilla chips with crispy baked farfalle pasta and let the real stars of the show, the spinach and artichokes, shine in a creamy low-calorie sauce. I have to admit that several times, instead of portioning out this recipe like I should and saving the rest for later, I have found myself leaning over the stove, scooping up spoonful after spoonful of this dip. It is highly addictive, so be sure to use a little calorie caution and stick to the portion size.

MAKES 8 SERVINGS

SPINACH ARTICHOKE DIP

One 12-ounce package soft silken tofu

¼ cup canola oil

½ teaspoon onion powder

¼ cup nutritional yeast

1 teaspoon fine sea salt

2 garlic cloves, chopped

One 10-ounce package frozen chopped spinach, thawed and water pressed out

One 14-ounce can artichoke hearts, drained and chopped

Freshly ground black pepper

FARFALLE CHIPS

1 cup plain almond milk

¼ cup Ener-G Egg Replacer

2 cups bow-tie (farfalle) pasta, cooked according to package directions

1 cup seasoned bread crumbs

1 teaspoon chili powder

¼ teaspoon fine sea salt

To make the dip:

Preheat the oven to 375°F. Spray a 2-quart casserole dish with nonstick cooking spray.

Put the tofu, oil, onion powder, nutritional yeast, salt, and

PER SERVING
(DIP ALONE):

119 Calories

7 g Protein

9 g Total fat

1 g Saturated fat

0 g Monounsaturated fat

10 g Carbohydrates

5 g Fiber

1 g Sugar

83 mg Calcium

2 mg Iron

359 mg Sodium

PER SERVING
(DIP AND FARFALLE CHIPS):

192 Calories

10 g Protein

9 g Total fat

1 g Saturated fat

0 g Monounsaturated fat

24 g Carbohydrates

5 g Fiber

1 g Sugar

99 mg Calcium

2 mg Iron

844 mg Sodium

garlic into a blender and blend until smooth. Transfer to a medium bowl and stir in the spinach, artichoke hearts, and black pepper to taste. Transfer the dip mixture into the prepared casserole dish and bake for 20 minutes or until the dip begins to bubble and is warmed through.

To make the chips:

Preheat the oven to 400°F and line a large baking sheet with nonstick foil or parchment paper.

Whisk together the milk and egg replacer in a medium bowl until thoroughly combined. Add the pasta and toss to coat.

Combine the bread crumbs, chili powder, and sea salt in a large sealable plastic bag. Drain the pasta then add it to bread crumb mixture and toss until completely coated. Arrange the coated pasta in a single layer on the prepared baking sheet. Spray with cooking spray and bake for 10 to 15 minutes or until golden and crisp.

sides

EVEN THOUGH THESE dishes are considered side dishes, there is no reason why they shouldn't be treated with the same fanfare as the main event. In fact, according to the USDA "My Plate" method of eating that was released in 2011, our side dishes should take a more prominent position on our plates, with half of the standard 9-inch plate filled with fruit and/or vegetables, one fourth of the plate filled with starch (like rice, pasta, potatoes, or breads) and the remaining one fourth with protein.

Five-Minute Garlic Spinach

MAKES 4 SERVINGS

It never ceases to amaze me how quickly a big bag of fresh spinach wilts down to just a couple cups in just minutes on the stove top. Still, I've grown to love the flavor of wilted or sautéed fresh spinach so much that I can't imagine eating that water-logged frozen variety ever again. I've scaled this recipe down to a 10-ounce bag of fresh baby spinach because most people don't have a pan that will accommodate a larger amount. However, if you happen to have a monster skillet hanging around the kitchen like I do, feel free to double the recipe—even if you were to eat 3 servings in one sitting you would barely break the 200-calorie mark—and really, can you ever have too much spinach in your life?

1 tablespoon extra virgin olive oil

1 small shallot, thinly sliced

5 garlic cloves, thinly sliced

10 ounces fresh baby spinach

¼ teaspoon fine sea salt

Warm the oil in a large skillet over medium heat. Add the shallot and garlic and sauté until garlic and shallots are both soft and fragrant. Add the spinach and cook until wilted, 2 to 3 minutes. Sprinkle with salt and toss. Serve warm.

PER SERVING:

67 Calories

3 g Protein

4 g Total fat

1 g Saturated fat

0 g Monounsaturated fat

7 g Carbohydrates

3 g Fiber

0 g Sugar

120 mg Calcium

2 mg Iron

218 mg Sodium

Braised Baby Bok Choy

I'm a little odd when it comes to bok choy. While baby bok choy is my best friend, full-size bok choy is my archnemesis. The tender, sweet leaves of bok choy are my favorite part, and the full-size version with its puny little leaves just doesn't cut it—there's way too much stem. It's nearly impossible to mess up a recipe that calls for baby bok choy. It has a wonderfully earthy, sweet flavor that can stand on its own, and it needs only the smallest amounts of lemon, ginger, and garlic to really come to life.

1 pound baby bok choy

1 tablespoon canola oil

½ teaspoon agave nectar

2 tablespoons water

1 teaspoon cornstarch

2 teaspoons lemon juice

1 tablespoon minced fresh ginger

1 garlic clove, minced

¼ cup sliced almonds

Roughly chop the bok choy and set aside. Warm the oil in a large braising pan over medium heat. While the oil is warming, whisk together the agave nectar, water, cornstarch, and lemon juice and set aside. Add the ginger and garlic to the braising pan and sauté until fragrant, about 30 seconds. Add the bok choy and cook until softened, about 2 minutes. Add the agave mixture and stir well. Cover the pan and continue to cook for an additional 2 minutes. Remove from the heat and fold in the almonds. Serve warm.

MAKES 4 SERVINGS

PER SERVING:

126 Calories

3 g Protein

8 g Total fat

1 g Saturated fat

5 g Monounsaturated fat

12 g Carbohydrates

2 g Fiber

1 g Sugar

55 mg Calcium

2 mg Iron

282 mg Sodium

Broccoli Casserole

MAKES 8 SERVINGS

As soon as I was able to reach the stove and stir a pot, I was cooking. Not everything I made was a culinary masterpiece, but I did my best with what my little childhood palate knew to make and experiment with. One such experiment was adding broccoli (and sometimes peas) to boxed macaroni and cheese to make myself a little broccoli casserole—a relatively standard dish, but at nine or ten years old I thought I was being pretty innovative. I've stepped it up a bit since my childhood introduction to the culinary classics, but I still can't resist the opportunity to toss some vegetables into mac and cheese. This is a takeoff on my traditional Macaroni and Cheese *recipe from* Quick and Easy Vegan Comfort Food *and* Quick and Easy Vegan Celebrations. *With its added broccoli and tomatoes, this filling casserole would blow my nine-year-old self's taste buds away.*

2½ cups spiral pasta

1 medium Yukon Gold potato, peeled and diced

½ medium carrot, peeled and diced

⅓ cup white or yellow onion, diced

1 garlic clove, chopped

1¼ cups water

¼ cup canola oil

⅓ cup raw cashews

1 teaspoon fine sea salt

⅛ teaspoon dry mustard

1 tablespoon fresh lemon juice

¼ teaspoon ground black pepper

2 cup chopped fresh or thawed broccoli

⅓ cup canned petite diced tomatoes

PER SERVING:

175 Calories

5 g Protein

10 g Total fat

1 g Saturated fat

0 g Monounsaturated fat

19 g Carbohydrates

3 g Fiber

3 g Sugar

36 mg Calcium

1 mg Iron

359 mg Sodium

Preheat the oven to 350°F. Spray a 2-quart casserole dish with nonstick cooking spray.

Prepare the pasta according to the package directions. Drain and set aside.

While the pasta is cooking, combine the potato, carrot,

onion, garlic, and water in a small saucepan. Bring to a boil, cover, and simmer for 10 minutes or until the vegetables are tender. (The smaller you cut the vegetables, the less time they will take to cook.)

Put the canola oil, cashews, salt, mustard, lemon juice, black pepper, and cooked vegetable mixture with their cooking water into a blender and blend until completely smooth.

Toss the cooked pasta well with the pureed sauce, broccoli, and tomatoes, then transfer to the prepared casserole dish. Bake for 30 minutes or until the cheese sauce bubbles.

Sesame Broccolini

MAKES 6 SERVINGS

Broccolini is not the easiest vegetable to find, and once you find it the next question is what to do with it. The tiny, flower-lined florets of broccolini are a bit sweeter than broccoli, with almost a hint of asparagus in the long stalks. I like to steam it very lightly, just enough to turn it a vibrant green, then toss it in this sweet, nutty balsamic and toasted sesame oil dressing. Serving it warm right out the steamer is my favorite way to preserve the crunch. Because too much heat will soften the vegetable and take away from its flavor, I don't recommend reheating your leftovers. However, you can eat them chilled the next day and they will be superb.

1 pound broccolini

2 tablespoons extra virgin olive oil

1 teaspoon toasted sesame oil

1 tablespoon balsamic vinegar

2 tablespoons orange juice

1 teaspoon Bragg Liquid Aminos

½ teaspoon onion powder

Steam the broccolini until tender, about 3 to 5 minutes. Meanwhile, whisk together the olive oil, sesame oil, vinegar, orange juice, liquid aminos, and onion powder in a medium bowl. Add the steamed broccolini and toss until coated. Serve warm.

PER SERVING:

76 Calories

2 g Protein

5 g Total fat

1 g Saturated fat

0 g Monounsaturated fat

6 g Carbohydrates

2 g Fiber

2 g Sugar

36 mg Calcium

1 mg Iron

79 mg Sodium

Gingered Brussels Sprouts

I grew up in a family of vegetable eaters. We never grumbled when green beans, carrots, collard greens, or zucchini was put in front of us; we just gobbled it all up. Brussels sprouts were no exception. I was intrigued by the little green ball of leaves and loved dissecting each sprout before I ate it (playing with food was not discouraged as long as we ate it when we were finished). Back then we kept it simple: steamed Brussels sprouts with a little margarine, salt, and pepper was about as fancy as it got. These Brussels sprouts, on the other hand, are a far cry from the sprouts of my youth, and they are one of the reasons fresh ginger is now a staple in my home. In fact, I've been known to increase the ginger to 2, or sometimes even 3 tablespoons.

1 pound fresh Brussels sprouts

1 teaspoon canola oil

1 tablespoon minced fresh ginger

½ teaspoon toasted sesame oil

2 teaspoons agave nectar

½ teaspoon fine sea salt

1 tablespoon vermouth

1 tablespoon sesame seeds

Quarter the Brussels sprouts and steam until tender, about 5 minutes. Meanwhile, warm the canola oil in a large skillet. Add the ginger and cook until soft and fragrant, about 1 minute. Whisk together the sesame oil, agave nectar, salt, vermouth, and sesame seeds and add to the skillet. Add Brussels sprouts and toss to coat. Serve warm.

MAKES 6 SERVINGS

PER SERVING:

60 Calories

2 g Protein

3 g Total fat

0 g Saturated fat

1 g Monounsaturated fat

8 g Carbohydrates

2 g Fiber

3 g Sugar

51 mg Calcium

1 mg Iron

213 mg Sodium

Refried Beans

The funny thing about refried beans is that they don't actually require any type of "refrying" at all. You can just take a big pot of seasoned pinto beans, in this case Pinto Beans in Ancho Chile Sauce, add a little oil and water, and you've got yourself a beautiful batch of protein-packed refried beans.

1 tablespoon extra virgin olive oil

1 tablespoon Ancho Chile Sauce (page 235)

1 recipe Pinto Beans in Ancho Chile Sauce (page 168)

½ cup water

Warm the oil in a medium saucepan over medium-high heat. Add the chile sauce and cook until fragrant, about 1 minute. Add the beans and water. Reduce the heat to medium and stir and mash the beans until smooth and thick, 5 to 10 minutes. Serve.

PER SERVING
(⅓ CUP):

187 Calories

7 g Protein

7 g Total fat

1 g Saturated fat

0 g Monounsaturated fat

25 g Carbohydrates

6 g Fiber

0 g Sugar

69 mg Calcium

3 mg Iron

898 mg Sodium

PER SERVING
(¼ CUP):

149 Calories

6 g Protein

6 g Total fat

1 g Saturated fat

0 g Monounsaturated fat

20 g Carbohydrates

5 g Fiber

0 g Sugar

55 mg Calcium

2 mg Iron

718 mg Sodium

Refried Black Beans

I've discovered something about making homemade versions of foods you normally find canned or only eat in restaurants—when you make them at home from scratch it gives the meal an instant wow factor. When your friends ask you how you made these refried beans, put on your most exasperated face and say, "I don't even know where to begin!" They'll immediately assume you have the chops of a professional chef, and the secret of how quick and easy these actually are will be between you, me, and the other readers of this book.

1 tablespoon extra virgin olive oil

2 tablespoons Ancho Chile Sauce (page 235)

2 cups cooked black beans

¼ teaspoon fine sea salt

½ cup vegetable stock

Warm the oil in a medium saucepan over medium-high heat. Add the chile sauce and cook until fragrant, about 1 minute. Add the beans, salt, and vegetable stock. Reduce the heat to medium and stir and mash the beans until smooth and thick, 5 to 10 minutes. Serve.

MAKES 1¼ CUPS

PER SERVING
(¼ CUP):

122 Calories

6 g Protein

3 g Total fat

0 g Saturated fat

0 g Monounsaturated fat

18 g Carbohydrates

6 g Fiber

0 g Sugar

22 mg Calcium

2 mg Iron

222 mg Sodium

Hoppin' John

No one really knows who Hoppin' John was. Some say the creator of this dish was a slave with a limp. Some say it's a mispronunciation of a dish whose real name is long lost in translation. One thing's for sure, though: its South Carolina origins make it a truly southern, stick-to-your-ribs classic. And it's packed with protein, fiber, and flavor, too.

1 tablespoon canola oil

½ cup diced sweet or Vidalia onion

½ large green bell pepper, diced

2 garlic cloves, minced

3 cups vegetable stock

½ teaspoon hickory liquid smoke

1 bay leaf

½ pound dried black-eyed peas

½ teaspoon sugar

2 cups cooked brown rice

Warm the oil in a skillet and add the onions and bell pepper. Sauté for 3 to 4 minutes until the onions are translucent. Add the garlic and sauté for an additional minute, being careful not to burn the garlic. Add the stock, liquid smoke, bay leaf, peas, and sugar. Bring to a low boil, reduce heat, cover, and simmer for 30 to 40 minutes until the peas are tender and most, but not all, of the liquid is absorbed. Remove the bay leaf. Add the cooked brown rice and stir to combine.

PER SERVING:

146 Calories

3 g Protein

3 g Total fat

0 g Saturated fat

0 g Monounsaturated fat

27 g Carbohydrates

4 g Fiber

4 g Sugar

61 mg Calcium

1 mg Iron

279 mg Sodium

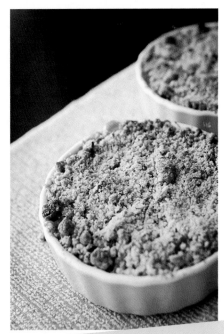

Sweet Potato Soufflé (page 122)

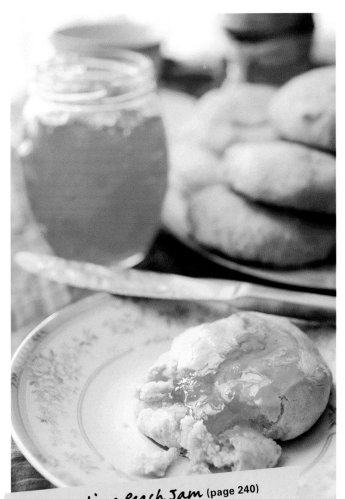

South Carolina Peach Jam (page 240)
on Buttermilk Biscuits (page 68)

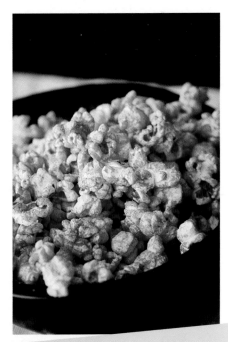

BBQ Popcorn (page 91)

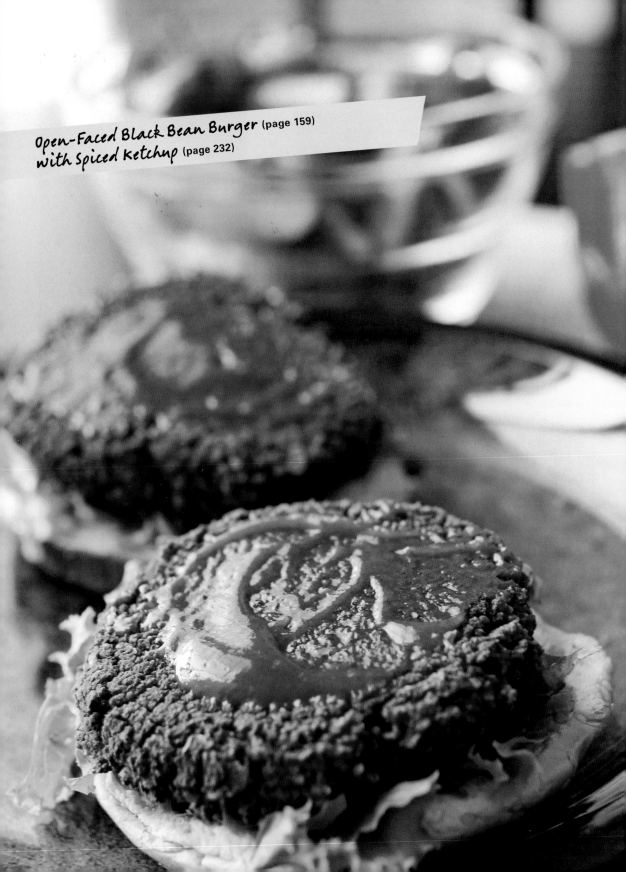

Open-Faced Black Bean Burger (page 159)
with Spiced Ketchup (page 232)

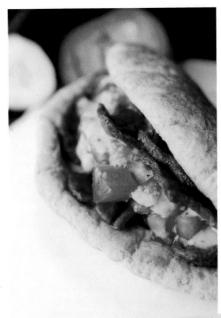

Gyros with Tzatziki Sauce (page 192)

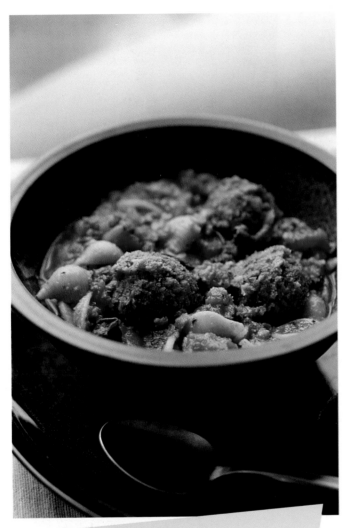

Meatball Soup (page 152)

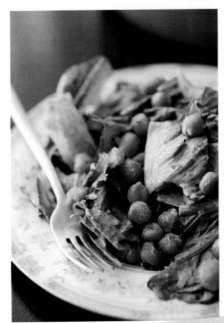

Caesar Salad with Chickpea Croutons (page 126)

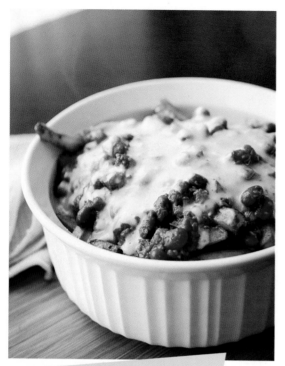

Chili Cheese Fries (page 165)

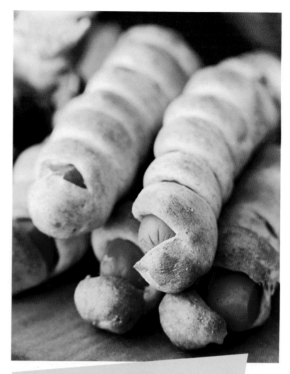

Corn Dogs (page 162)

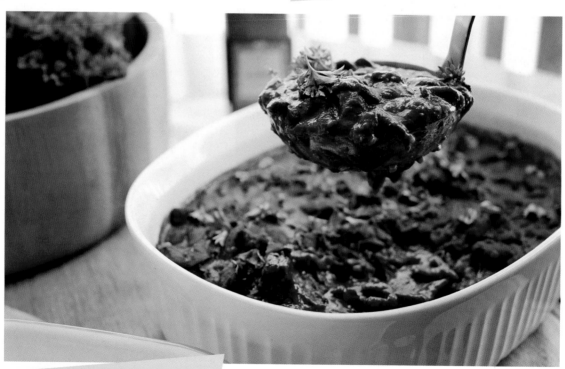

Cincinnati Chili (page 170)

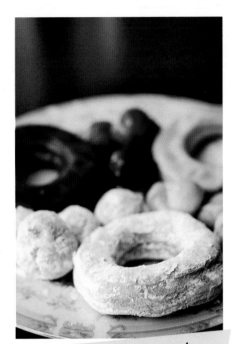

Moon Dusted Donuts and Glazed Donuts (pages 214–15)

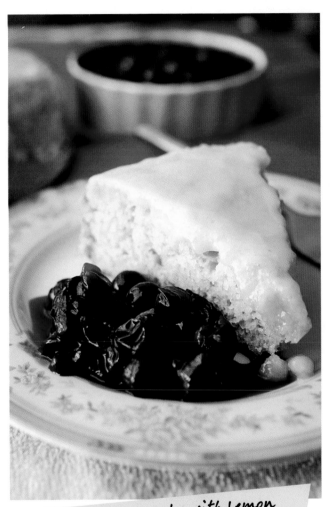

Lemon Cornmeal Cake with Lemon Glaze and Blueberry Sauce (page 212)

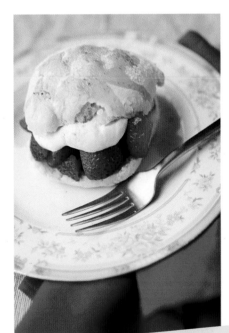

Strawberry Shortcakes with Balsamic Syrup (page 208)

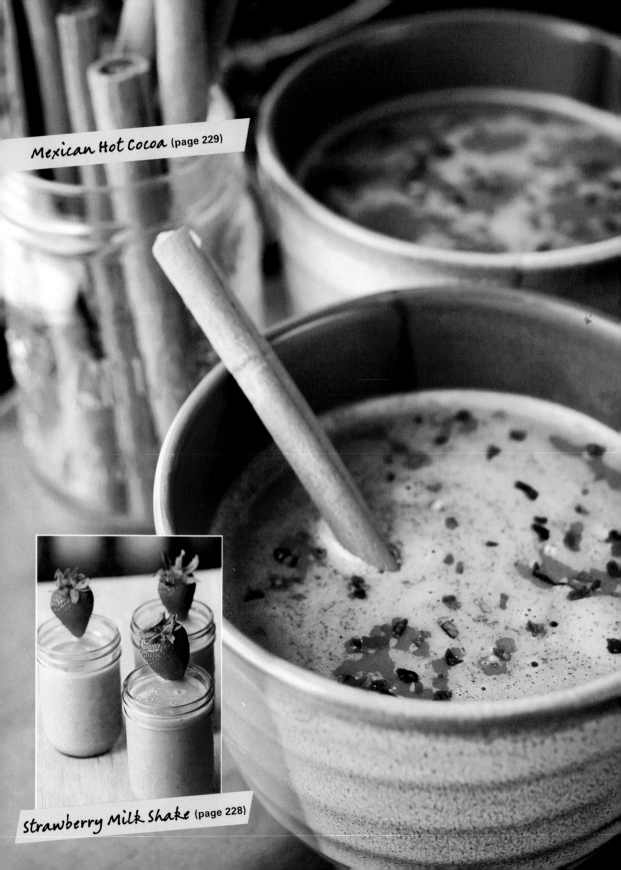

Mexican Hot Cocoa (page 229)

Strawberry Milk Shake (page 228)

Mexican Rice

Many people mistakenly think that rice that has color, such as Mexican rice, Spanish rice, or yellow rice, is a whole-grain product because the rice is not visibly white. However, all these preparations are just white rice with seasonings, so they don't contain the additional protein, fiber, and minerals that whole-grain brown rice does. You may think that brown rice is a pain to cook, but the good news is that quick-cooking brown rice cooks up as fast as white rice while packing a big nutritional punch.

MAKES 8 SERVINGS

1 large very ripe tomato

1 medium white onion

2 tablespoons canola oil

4 garlic cloves, minced

2 medium jalapeños, seeds discarded and flesh minced

⅓ cup vegetable stock

½ cup water

1 tablespoon ketchup

½ teaspoon fine sea salt

1¾ cups quick-cooking brown rice

Put the tomato and onion into a food processor and puree until smooth. Warm the canola oil in a medium saucepan over medium heat. Add the garlic and jalapeños and cook for 1 to 2 minutes until fragrant. Stir in the pureed tomato mixture, vegetable stock, water, ketchup, and sea salt and bring to a boil. Add the brown rice and cook until all the liquid is absorbed and the rice is tender, about 15 minutes.

PER SERVING:

196 Calories

4 g Protein

5 g Total fat

0 g Saturated fat

0 g Monounsaturated fat

35 g Carbohydrates

2 g Fiber

2 g Sugar

23 mg Calcium

1 mg Iron

195 mg Sodium

Zucchini Fritters

MAKES 12 FRITTERS

Whether you bake these or fry them, whether you use oil or nonstick cooking spray—at 35 to 55 calories a fritter, you can munch on these guilt free.

1 pound zucchini, grated

½ teaspoon fine sea salt

¼ cup shredded carrot

1 teaspoon dried parsley

1 garlic clove, minced

¼ teaspoon ground black pepper

½ cup plain soy yogurt

½ cup unbleached all-purpose flour

2 tablespoons canola oil, optional

PER FRITTER
(WITH CANOLA OIL):

55 Calories

1 g Protein

3 g Total fat

0 g Saturated fat

0 g Monounsaturated fat

7 g Carbohydrates

1 g Fiber

2 g Sugar

27 mg Calcium

0 mg Iron

105 mg Sodium

PER FRITTER
(WITH NONSTICK COOKING SPRAY, PAN-FRIED OR BAKED):

35 Calories

1 g Protein

0 g Total fat

0 g Saturated fat

0 g Monounsaturated fat

7 g Carbohydrates

1 g Fiber

2 g Sugar

27 mg Calcium

0 mg Iron

105 mg Sodium

Thoroughly combine the grated zucchini, salt, carrot, parsley, garlic, black pepper, and yogurt in a large bowl. Add the flour and stir until completely combined.

Directions for pan-frying

Warm a skillet over medium to medium-high heat and add the canola oil or spray with nonstick cooking spray. Form a little less than ¼ cup of the zucchini mixture into a ball and carefully drop into the oil. Repeat with the remaining zucchini mixture, leaving about 1½ inches between each ball, then flatten each fritter with a spatula. Fry until golden on both sides, about 3 to 4 minutes per side.

Directions for baking

Preheat the oven to 425°F. Line a baking sheet with nonstick foil or parchment paper and spray with nonstick cooking spray.

Form a little less than ¼ cup of the zucchini mixture into a ball and place on the prepared baking sheet. Repeat with the remaining zucchini mixture, arranging the balls in a single layer on the baking sheet with about 1½ inches between them. Flatten each fritter with a spatula then spray with cooking spray. Bake until the fritters are golden and crisp around edges, about 30 minutes.

Fried Green Tomatoes

MAKES 8 SERVINGS

There are some things that just aren't the same without a little oil in them, and fried green tomatoes is one of them. I wouldn't dare disturb this southern classic by baking it or using cooking spray to pan fry it. Besides, at only 178 calories per serving, why kick out the canola oil? I do have a little flavor combination that I love that is anything but southern: a dollop of Tzatziki Sauce (page 192) on each fried tomato is irresistibly good. Shhh . . . the southern cooking police never have to know.

¼ cup canola oil

¾ cup cornmeal

¾ cup unbleached all-purpose flour

1 tablespoon garlic powder

¼ teaspoon cayenne

½ cup unsweetened plain soy yogurt

1 cup water

3 large green tomatoes, cut into ¼-inch slices

Warm the canola oil over medium heat in a large skillet. While the oil is warming, combine the cornmeal, flour, garlic powder, and cayenne in a shallow bowl. Whisk together the yogurt and water in another shallow bowl. Dip the tomato slices in the yogurt mixture then press into the cornmeal mixture, coating on all sides.

Fry the breaded tomato slices in small batches in the skillet until crispy and golden brown, about 2 to 3 minutes on each side. Allow to drain on paper towels.

PER SERVING:

178 Calories

4 g Protein

8 g Total fat

1 g Saturated fat

0 g Monounsaturated fat

24 g Carbohydrates

2 g Fiber

3 g Sugar

44 mg Calcium

2 mg Iron

12 mg Sodium

Eggplant Fries

I have a love-hate relationship with eggplant that extends back to the '80s. However, I discovered there's one way that I always like eggplant, and that's breaded and baked (or fried) with a little marinara sauce. Whether it's Eggplant Parmesan (page 183) or these Eggplant Fries, if you bread it I'll eat it. This, by the way, is a great go-to method for satisfying the picky eaters in your life. This recipe is a testament to the fact that just because something is breaded doesn't mean it's full of calories. These fries are packed with big-time flavor, but at 85 calories a serving, they barely put a dent in your calorie requirement for the day. Eat Eggplant Fries with ketchup as you would traditional fries or dip them in marinara sauce.

MAKES 8 SERVINGS

1¼ cups unbleached all-purpose flour

½ teaspoon Old Bay seasoning

¼ teaspoon ground black pepper

1 cup plain almond milk

1 pound eggplant, peeled and cut into fries

Preheat the oven to 425°F. Coat a baking sheet with nonstick cooking spray.

Combine the flour, Old Bay seasoning, and black pepper in a medium shallow dish. Put milk in a separate small shallow dish. In small batches, dip the eggplant pieces in the milk then press into the flour mixture to cover and lay out in rows on the prepared baking sheet. When all the eggplant fries have been breaded, spray with nonstick cooking spray.

Bake for approximately 10 to 15 minutes then carefully turn the fries. Bake for another 10 to 15 minutes until golden brown.

PER SERVING:

85 Calories

3 g Protein

0 g Total fat

0 g Saturated fat

0 g Monounsaturated fat

18 g Carbohydrates

2 g Fiber

1 g Sugar

8 mg Calcium

1 mg Iron

87 mg Sodium

Cheese Fries

I know cheese fries are supposed to be a side item, but I am guilty of eating them as a full meal. What never ceases to surprise me about this recipe is how filling it is. I've sat down to an Open-Faced Black Bean Burger with Spiced Ketchup (page 159) and a side of Cheese Fries, and I was so stuffed afterward I could barely move! The best part about that hearty meal of burger and fries slathered in cheese sauce is that it yields a total of only 382 calories. To put that in perspective, the average 4-ounce fast food cheeseburger has over 300 calories in the burger alone. Isn't being vegan fantastic?! Of course, if you're in the mood for something even lighter, you can leave out the cheese and eat the fries plain, as pictured on the cover, for just 98 calories per serving.

3 large russet potatoes, scrubbed and cut into ¼- to ½-inch-thick strips

1½ tablespoons canola oil

½ teaspoon fine sea salt

¼ teaspoon paprika

1 recipe Classic Cheese Sauce (page 237)

Preheat the oven to 450°F and line a baking sheet with nonstick foil or parchment paper.

Toss the potatoes with the oil in a large bowl. Add the salt and paprika and toss again.

Arrange the potatoes on the baking sheet in a single layer. Bake for 30 minutes or until golden brown and crispy. Divide the fries among 6 serving plates and top with Classic Cheese Sauce.

PER SERVING:

187 Calories

4 g Protein

8 g Total fat

0 g Saturated fat

0 g Monounsaturated fat

26 g Carbohydrates

4 g Fiber

1 g Sugar

25 mg Calcium

2 mg Iron

506 mg Sodium

Corn Pudding

I was turned on to the concept of corn pudding last winter by my grandmother, who wanted to, in her words, "make a meal with no fuss" at Christmas. Incidentally, "no fuss" in her world apparently means a five-course meal—at least I know where my cooking genes came from! My grandmother's recipe was so far from vegan I didn't dare try to replicate it. Instead, I decided to create a corn pudding recipe of my very own, and I think my version would make her proud.

2½ cups fresh white or yellow corn kernels, from about 3 ears

2 tablespoons unbleached all-purpose flour

2 tablespoons sugar

½ teaspoon fine sea salt

¼ teaspoon ground black pepper

⅛ teaspoon cayenne

2 tablespoons Earth Balance margarine, softened

½ cup pureed soft silken tofu or unsweetened plain soy yogurt

1 cup plain almond milk

Preheat the oven to 325°F. Spray a 2-quart baking dish with nonstick cooking spray.

Put ½ cup of the corn kernels, the flour, sugar, salt, black pepper, cayenne, margarine, and tofu into a blender and blend until smooth. Transfer the mixture to a medium bowl and stir in the remaining 2 cups corn kernels and the milk. Pour into the prepared baking dish and bake for 40 to 45 minutes until a knife is inserted into the center comes out clean. Serve warm.

PER SERVING:

130 Calories

3 g Protein

5 g Total fat

2 g Saturated fat

0 g Monounsaturated fat

21 g Carbohydrates

2 g Fiber

7 g Sugar

45 mg Calcium

1 mg Iron

241 mg Sodium

Sweet Potato Soufflé 📷

The best way to make this soufflé is by baking it in individual ramekins to ensure that you stay within the 8-serving portion size. In truth, this is such a sweet and rich dish you can probably split each serving in half. If you're like me, though—crazy about sweet potatoes—that will probably be impossible. I don't blame you!

PER SERVING:

346 Calories
5 g Protein
15 g Total fat
3 g Saturated fat
7 g Monounsaturated fat
51 g Carbohydrates
3 g Fiber
26 g Sugar
105 mg Calcium
2 mg Iron
296 mg Sodium

If you're using ramekins you will have lots of leftover topping, so feel free to reduce the topping by half. Here's the nutrition info if you use half the topping:

PER SERVING:

240 Calories
4 g Protein
8 g Total fat
1 g Saturated fat
3 g Monounsaturated fat
41 g Carbohydrates
2 g Fiber
20 g Sugar
81 mg Calcium
2 mg Iron
221 mg Sodium

SOUFFLÉ

3 cups baked and mashed garnet sweet potatoes (about 3 medium potatoes)
¼ cup granulated sugar
½ cup plain soy yogurt
½ cup plain almond milk
1 teaspoon vanilla extract
¼ teaspoon fine sea salt

TOPPING

½ cup light brown sugar
½ cup self-rising flour
3 tablespoons Earth Balance margarine, softened
1 cup chopped pecans

To make the soufflé:

Preheat the oven to 400°F. Spray an 8-inch square baking dish or eight 4-ounce ramekins with nonstick cooking spray.

Combine the sweet potatoes, granulated sugar, yogurt, milk, vanilla, and salt. Transfer the mixture to the baking dish or divide evenly among the ramekins.

To make the topping:

Combine brown sugar and flour. With a pastry cutter or fork, incorporate the margarine into the sugar mixture; the mixture will look crumbly. Add the pecans and stir well to combine.

Sprinkle the topping over the sweet potato mixture. Bake for 20 to 25 minutes until the topping is golden brown.

Spiced Cranberry Sauce

Even though cranberry sauce is technically a sauce, I never used to use it that way. I'd typically eat it all by itself, enjoying every bit of its sweet tartness. While experimenting in the kitchen one day I decided to add one of my favorite combinations of spice blends (mace, allspice, and ginger) to a pot of simmering cranberry sauce and see what happened. What happened was a transformation of cranberry sauce from a very good side dish into a phenomenal side dish, spread, and all-purpose sauce. Now I eat Spiced Cranberry Sauce instead of gravy on everything from Sweet Potato Drop Biscuits (page 71) to Chik'n-Fried Seitan (page 194). I use it as a sandwich spread, and I've even added a couple spoonfuls to top off a bowl of Vanilla-Almond Ice Cream (page 201). These serving sizes are pretty generous, so if you're using it as a sauce or spread instead of a side dish, you will probably use half the amount, reducing the calories to less than 50 for this tart and sweet treat.

One 10-ounce package fresh or frozen cranberries

½ cup sugar

⅓ cup orange juice

⅔ cup water

1 cinnamon stick

⅛ teaspoon ground nutmeg or mace

⅛ teaspoon ground allspice

⅛ teaspoon ground ginger

Bring the cranberries, sugar, orange juice, water, cinnamon stick, nutmeg, allspice, and ginger to a boil in a 2-quart saucepan, stirring occasionally. Reduce the heat, cover, and simmer for 10 minutes, stirring occasionally.

Uncover and cook for an additional 10 minutes. Remove from the heat, remove the cinnamon stick if desired, and allow to cool. The sauce will thicken as it cools.

PER SERVING:

93 Calories

0 g Protein

0 g Total fat

0 g Saturated fat

0 g Monounsaturated fat

24 g Carbohydrates

2 g Fiber

19 g Sugar

6 mg Calcium

0 mg Iron

2 mg Sodium

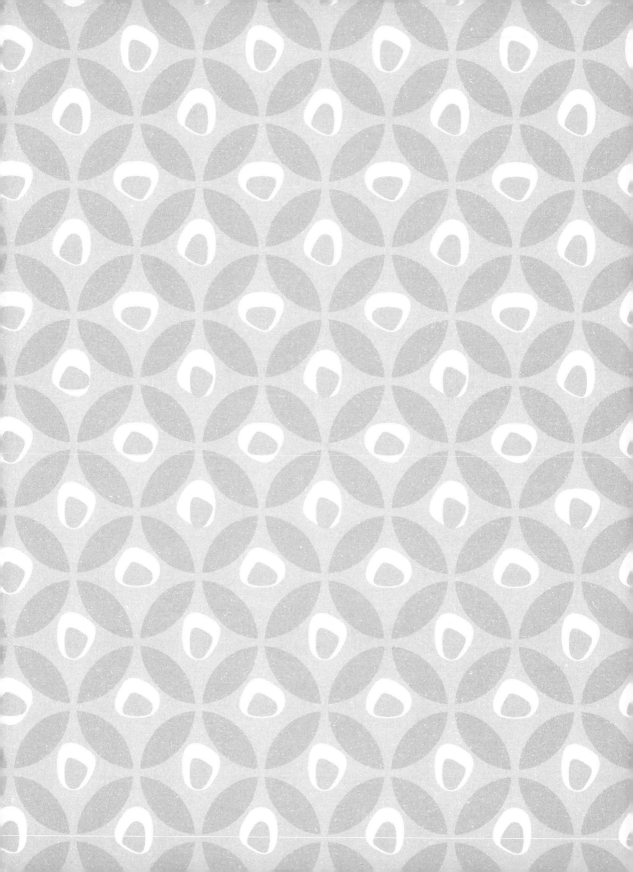

The Salad Bar

OFTEN WHEN I tell people that I'm vegan the reply is, "I'd go vegan but I don't like salads." Somehow, over the years, salads have become synonymous with a plant-based diet and healthy eating. However, as you can see from this book, a plant-based diet is full of rich, filling comfort foods, not just salads. I, for one, am guilty of straying away from eating salads in public because of the image that vegans only eat rabbit food. But with hearty, filling salads like Caesar Salad with Chickpea Croutons, Spiced Moroccan Salad with Ancho-Agave Pecans, and Sweet Potato Salad, I can munch my rabbit food proudly to the envy of all who see it!

Caesar Salad with Chickpea Croutons 📷

MAKES 4 SERVINGS

There's no rule that says croutons have to be made from bread, or if the rule does exist then I would like to submit this recipe as my appeal to overturn it immediately! What better way to add a little punch of protein to a traditional Caesar salad than by sprinkling garlicky, crisp chickpea croutons on top? This salad packs in 12 grams of protein per serving as well as nearly 17 percent of the recommended daily value of iron. Not too shabby for a salad.

CHICKPEA CROUTONS

2 cups cooked chickpeas

¼ teaspoon garlic powder

½ teaspoon fine sea salt

2 teaspoons canola oil

CAESAR DRESSING

3 tablespoons fresh lemon juice

½ teaspoon Dijon mustard

1 tablespoon capers

1 garlic clove, chopped

3 tablespoons nutritional yeast

¼ teaspoon vegan Worcestershire sauce

¼ teaspoon fine sea salt

¼ teaspoon ground white pepper

½ cup unsweetened plain soy yogurt

1 tablespoon extra virgin olive oil

2 heads romaine, washed, dried, and thinly sliced

PER SERVING:

208 Calories

12 g Protein

9 g Total fat

1 g Saturated fat

0 g Monounsaturated fat

28 g Carbohydrates

8 g Fiber

5 g Sugar

113 mg Calcium

3 mg Iron

533 mg Sodium

To make the croutons:

Preheat the oven to 400°F and line a baking sheet with nonstick foil or parchment paper.

Put all the crouton ingredients into a medium bowl and toss to coat. Spread the coated chickpeas in single layer on the prepared baking sheet and bake for 25 to 30 minutes until lightly browned and crispy. Store in an airtight container for up to 2 weeks.

To make the dressing:

Put lemon juice, Dijon mustard, capers, garlic, nutritional yeast, Worcestershire sauce, salt, white pepper, and yogurt into a blender and blend until smooth and creamy. Turn the blender down to its lowest speed and slowly add the oil until fully incorporated.

Put the lettuce into a large bowl then add the Caesar Dressing and toss until every leaf is coated. Transfer the salad to serving plates and divide Chickpea Croutons evenly among salads.

Chef's Salad

MAKES 4 SERVINGS

A green salad is just a green salad. You can add as many vegetables, nuts, seeds, fruits, or different types of lettuce as you like, but ultimately it's just salad. What really sets one salad apart from the other is the dressing. A Caesar salad with Thousand Island dressing on it definitely wouldn't be a Caesar salad, and for me, a Chef's Salad isn't a Chef's Salad without the perfect French dressing. Resist the temptation to reach for a bottled brand and whip up a batch of homemade Frenchy Dressing instead. It'll turn a regular ole salad into a masterpiece.

1 pound green leaf lettuce

1 small cucumber, peeled and cut into thin slices

½ cup sliced radishes

1 medium tomato, chopped

1 small scallion, thinly sliced

1 medium carrot, peeled and grated

1 recipe Roasted Tofu (page 38)

½ cup Frenchy Dressing (page 239)

Arrange the salad ingredients on 4 serving plates, dividing the ingredients evenly between them. Chill, then drizzle with the dressing right before serving.

PER SERVING:

246 Calories

13 g Protein

14 g Total fat

2 g Saturated fat

0 g Monounsaturated fat

18 g Carbohydrates

5 g Fiber

9 g Sugar

156 mg Calcium

3 mg Iron

201 mg Sodium

Waldorf Salad

The Waldorf salad originated at the Waldorf Hotel back in the late 1800s, and until recently, I thought of it as a dish that should have stayed in the 1800s. Although I hadn't tried it, I just couldn't imagine the flavor combination of apples, celery, mayonnaise, and whipping cream to be any good. Then I was required to take a food production class for my master's in nutrition, and suddenly I found myself staring down a Waldorf salad recipe. I decided that there's no time like the present to veganize it, so I gave it a try. I'm so happy I did! The salad is sweet, crunchy, and not all "mayonnaisy" like I thought it would be.

½ cup nondairy whipping cream

1 tablespoon plus 1½ teaspoons agave nectar

1 pound gala apples, cored and diced

¼ cup plus 1 tablespoon pineapple juice

⅔ cup vegan mayonnaise

2 celery stalks, diced

3 tablespoons chopped walnuts

Chill a mixing bowl, the whipping cream, and the agave nectar for at least 30 minutes prior to preparing.

Toss the apples and pineapple juice in a large bowl, making sure the juice coats all the apples, and set aside.

Beat the whipping cream and agave nectar with an electric mixer until stiff peaks form. Fold in the mayonnaise. Drain the pineapple juice from the apples and toss with the celery and chopped walnuts to combine. Fold in just enough cream mixture to coat salad. Chill until ready to eat.

MAKES 8 SERVINGS

PER SERVING:

235 Calories

1 g Protein

17 g Total fat

3 g Saturated fat

0 g Monounsaturated fat

17 g Carbohydrates

1 g Fiber

12 g Sugar

15 mg Calcium

0 mg Iron

131 mg Sodium

Taco Salad

MAKES 4 SERVINGS

I'm a California girl through and through. No matter where I live, you simply can't take my love for Mexican food away from me. It is my definition of comfort food. I know that "salad" and "comfort food" don't usually appear in the same sentence, but all it takes is a little cumin, chili powder, lime, and cilantro for me to feel I'm home again.

DRESSING

⅓ cup chopped fresh cilantro

½ cup unsweetened plain soy yogurt

1 chipotle pepper in adobo sauce, minced

1 teaspoon ground cumin

1 teaspoon chili powder

2 teaspoons fresh lime juice

¼ teaspoon fine sea salt

4 cups shredded romaine lettuce

1 cup cherry tomatoes, halved

½ avocado, diced

½ small red onion, thinly sliced

1½ cups cooked black beans

1 cup steamed corn

PER SERVING:

200 Calories

10 g Protein

5 g Total fat

1 g Saturated fat

0 g Monounsaturated fat

32 g Carbohydrates

10 g Fiber

3 g Sugar

117 mg Calcium

3 mg Iron

168 mg Sodium

To make the dressing:

Combine all the dressing ingredients in a small bowl, cover, and refrigerate until ready to use, up to 2 days.

Combine all the salad ingredients in a large bowl. Drizzle with the dressing and toss to coat. Divide among 4 serving plates and serve immediately.

Creamy Coleslaw

There is simply no reason to buy a full head of cabbage and spend your afternoon shredding it down to fine ribbons to make the perfect coleslaw. Premade coleslaw mix has a fantastic blend of red and green cabbage and shredded carrots and is usually cheaper than buying the head of cabbage alone.

MAKES 8 SERVINGS

1 pound premade coleslaw mix

⅔ cup unsweetened plain soy yogurt

2 tablespoons unsweetened plain soy milk

2 tablespoons white vinegar

¼ cup sugar

½ teaspoon fine sea salt

Freshly ground black pepper

Combine all ingredients in a large bowl, cover with plastic wrap, and chill for at least 2 hours, preferably overnight.

PER SERVING:

50 Calories

2 g Protein

1 g Total fat

0 g Saturated fat

0 g Monounsaturated fat

11 g Carbohydrates

2 g Fiber

9 g Sugar

73 mg Calcium

0 mg Iron

164 mg Sodium

Spicy Kale Slaw

Running your eyes down this list of ingredients you might think I've gone a little mad, but just trust me on this one. I promise you, the combination of flavors is extraordinary. So it's time for your spice cabinet to flex its muscles and show us what it's made of!

It never ceases to amaze me how just ⅛ teaspoon of the right spice can change the entire flavor profile of a dish. Be sure to keep that in mind when adding the cayenne. Even if you're a big fan of spice I recommend starting off with ⅛ teaspoon of cayenne. The longer this slaw sits, the more the flavors develop, so if you overdo the cayenne you can go from having a subtly spicy slaw on Monday to a five-alarm fire in your mouth on Tuesday.

4 cups thinly sliced kale, any variety

1 medium carrot, peeled and grated

½ cup chopped pecans

¼ cup golden raisins

½ cup unsweetened plain soy yogurt

1 tablespoon apple cider vinegar

2 tablespoons sugar

½ teaspoon ground allspice

½ teaspoon dried oregano

½ teaspoon dried thyme

½ teaspoon paprika

⅛ to ¼ teaspoon cayenne

¼ teaspoon curry powder

¼ teaspoon fine sea salt

¼ teaspoon ground black pepper

⅛ teaspoon ground nutmeg

⅛ teaspoon ground cinnamon

⅛ teaspoon ground cloves

Put all the ingredients into a large bowl and toss until the kale is evenly coated. Cover and chill for at least an hour.

PER SERVING:

213 Calories

6 g Protein

11 g Total fat

1 g Saturated fat

6 g Monounsaturated fat

27 g Carbohydrates

5 g Fiber

16 g Sugar

185 mg Calcium

2 mg Iron

500 mg Sodium

Toasted Sesame Napa Cabbage Salad

When I say that you need a large bowl to combine the ingredients in this salad, I mean you need the largest bowl in your arsenal. As you start to cut the Napa cabbage you'll understand why. That little head of cabbage turns into a mountain of soft green curls almost big enough to create a replica of the iceberg that the Titanic hit.

1 head Napa cabbage, sliced thin

1 large carrot, peeled and shredded

2 scallions, thinly sliced

½ cup sliced almonds

3 tablespoons Bragg Liquid Aminos

1 tablespoon apple cider vinegar

2 garlic cloves, minced

½ teaspoon ground ginger

2 teaspoons toasted sesame oil

3 tablespoons agave nectar

Toss the cabbage, carrot, scallions, and almonds together in a large bowl. Whisk together the liquid aminos, vinegar, garlic, ginger, sesame oil, and agave nectar in a small bowl and pour over cabbage mixture. Toss to coat the cabbage evenly. Cover and chill for at least an hour, up to overnight.

MAKES 8 SERVINGS

PER SERVING:

104 Calories

3 g Protein

6 g Total fat

1 g Saturated fat

0 g Monounsaturated fat

12 g Carbohydrates

1 g Fiber

7 g Sugar

53 mg Calcium

1 mg Iron

381 mg Sodium

Roasted Fingerling Potato Salad

MAKES 4 SERVINGS

Fingerling potatoes are becoming easier and easier to find in conventional grocery stores. Not only that, but they are popping up in an assortment of colors, perfect for a fresh and tangy potato salad. I like to mix white, purple, and orange potatoes to create a stunning presentation.

1 pound fingerling potatoes, scrubbed and halved lengthwise

1 teaspoon extra virgin olive oil

⅛ teaspoon fine sea salt

1 tablespoon red wine vinegar

2 tablespoons flax oil

¾ teaspoon Dijon mustard

½ teaspoon celery salt

1 teaspoon dried tarragon

Preheat the oven to 450°F and line a baking sheet with nonstick foil or parchment paper.

Toss the potatoes in the oil and sprinkle with salt. Spread out on the prepared baking sheet and roast until tender, about 20 to 25 minutes. While the potatoes are roasting stir together vinegar, oil, mustard, celery salt, and tarragon.

Allow the cooked potatoes to cool completely. Toss with the vinegar mixture.

PER SERVING:

165 Calories

3 g Protein

8 g Total fat

1 g Saturated fat

0 g Monounsaturated fat

20 g Carbohydrates

1 g Fiber

0 g Sugar

3 mg Calcium

1 mg Iron

91 mg Sodium

Sweet Potato Salad

For some reason I only eat potato salad in the summer, and only with cookout-style foods like corn on the cob, baked beans, and sandwiches dripping with barbecue sauce, like the Carolina BBQ Sammich (page 160). It just doesn't feel right to eat traditional potato salad outside of this box, but sweet potato salad is a whole different ball game. I like to wait until autumn when sweet potatoes are in season and pair this salad with a spicy dish like Spicy Kale Slaw (page 132) or Chipotle Butternut Squash Bisque (page 146). Maybe one day I'll branch out and eat this salad in the summer or traditional potato salad in the fall, but I don't think it'll be anytime soon.

MAKES 6 SERVINGS

1½ pounds garnet sweet potatoes (about 1 large or 2 medium)

¼ cup golden raisins

⅓ cup unsweetened plain soy yogurt

1 tablespoon light brown sugar

1 scallion, thinly sliced

½ teaspoon garam masala

¼ teaspoon ground coriander

¼ teaspoon ground allspice

Put the potatoes into a medium stockpot with a pinch of sea salt and enough water to cover them by an inch. Bring to a boil and simmer until tender, about 20 minutes. Drain and let cool completely.

Combine the cooled potatoes with the raisins, yogurt, sugar, scallion, garam masala, coriander, and allspice in a medium bowl. Chill before serving.

PER SERVING:

169 Calories

3 g Protein

1 g Total fat

0 g Saturated fat

0 g Monounsaturated fat

40 g Carbohydrates

5 g Fiber

7 g Sugar

52 mg Calcium

1 mg Iron

13 mg Sodium

Moroccan Carrot Salad

MAKES 8 SERVINGS

The best way to make this salad is to grate the carrots with the grating blade of a food processor. Flip the blade over to the slicing edge and slice the shallot into thin, uniform slices, then toss all the ingredients together. Taking advantage of modern technology will cut your prep time down from 15 or 20 minutes to only 5.

½ teaspoon ground cumin

½ teaspoon ground ginger

¼ teaspoon ground cinnamon

¼ teaspoon ground coriander

¼ teaspoon cayenne

¼ teaspoon ground allspice

3 tablespoons extra virgin olive oil

2 tablespoons agave nectar

3 tablespoons fresh lemon juice

1 pound carrots, peeled and grated

1 small shallot, thinly sliced

Combine the cumin, ginger, cinnamon, coriander, cayenne, and allspice in a small bowl and set aside. Whisk together the oil, agave nectar, and lemon juice in a separate small bowl.

Put the carrots and shallot into a large bowl, add the spice blend and oil mixture, and toss to coat. Chill for at least 30 minutes.

PER SERVING:

93 Calories

1 g Protein

5 g Total fat

1 g Saturated fat

0 g Monounsaturated fat

12 g Carbohydrates

2 g Fiber

7 g Sugar

25 mg Calcium

0 mg Iron

41 mg Sodium

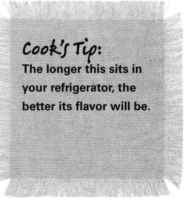

Cook's Tip:
The longer this sits in your refrigerator, the better its flavor will be.

Spiced Moroccan Salad
with Ancho-Agave Pecans

There are so many spices in this salad your taste buds won't know which way to turn, but I can guarantee that, no matter what direction they settle on, they will be happy.

MAKES 8 SERVINGS

ANCHO-AGAVE PECANS

½ cup agave nectar

1 tablespoon sugar

1 teaspoon ancho chile powder

2 cups pecan halves

8 cups mixed baby greens

4 cups Moroccan Carrot Salad (page 136)

To prepare the pecans:

Line a baking sheet with parchment paper. Bring agave, sugar, and chile powder to a boil in large, heavy skillet and stir until the sugar is dissolved. Add the pecans and cook, stirring often, until the syrup darkens and thickens, about 5 minutes. Turn out onto the prepared baking sheet. Separate the nuts using two forks. Cool completely and break the nuts apart before serving.

Divide the greens into 8 servings then top each with ½ cup carrot salad and ¼ cup Ancho-Agave Pecans.

PER SERVING:

334 Calories

4 g Protein

23 g Total fat

2 g Saturated fat

0 g Monounsaturated fat

34 g Carbohydrates

5 g Fiber

26 g Sugar

61 mg Calcium

2 mg Iron

55 mg Sodium

Millet Tabbouleh

Sometimes comfort foods are the familiar dishes we grew up eating as children, and sometimes they are foods we learn to love as adults, like this tabbouleh. I wasn't introduced to tabbouleh until my early twenties and now I don't know how I ever lived without it. It is downright shocking how just ¾ cup of millet will make 8 generous portions of tabbouleh. Try to use flax oil if you can; omega-3 fatty acids are an essential part of the diet, and this salad is a fantastic way to sneak some in.

1 teaspoon canola oil

¾ cup millet

1¾ cup water

1 cup chopped fresh parsley

4 scallions, chopped

1 medium tomato, chopped

1 medium lemon, juiced

¼ cup flax oil or extra virgin olive oil

⅛ teaspoon chili powder

Warm the oil in a medium saucepan over medium heat. Add the millet and toast for 2 minutes. Add the water and bring to a boil. Reduce the heat to low, cover, and cook until all the water has been absorbed, about 15 minutes. Take the pan off the heat and let stand, still covered, for 5 minutes. Uncover and allow the millet to cool completely.

Fluff the cooled millet with a fork then transfer to a medium bowl. Add the parsley, scallions, tomato, lemon juice, oil, and chili powder and toss until well combined. Chill for at least an hour.

PER SERVING:

146 Calories

3g Protein

8 g Total fat

1 g Saturated fat

2 g Monounsaturated fat

16 g Carbohydrates

2 g Fiber

1 g Sugar

21 mg Calcium

1 mg Iron

9 mg Sodium

Amaranth-Quinoa Salad

Amaranth is such a beautiful, flavorful grain that for centuries poets and writers have not been able to stop gushing about it. You can even find it referenced in Aesop's Fables. Amaranth is gluten-free, so if you've looked high and low and can't find it anywhere, try the gluten-free section of your grocery store.

2 cups vegetable stock

¾ cup quinoa, rinsed

½ cup amaranth

¼ cup fresh lemon juice

2 tablespoons flax oil

1 tablespoon fresh basil

1 tablespoon nutritional yeast

½ teaspoon dried oregano

1 garlic clove, minced

½ cup diced red bell pepper

½ cup diced cucumber

1 scallion, chopped

Bring the vegetable stock to a boil in a medium saucepan. Stir in the quinoa and amaranth then reduce the heat to low and cover. Cook until all the liquid is absorbed, about 10 minutes. While the grains are cooking, whisk together lemon juice, flax oil, basil, nutritional yeast, and oregano.

When the grains are cooked, transfer to a large bowl. Add the lemon juice mixture and the garlic, bell pepper, cucumber, and scallion and toss to combine. Chill for at least an hour before serving.

PER SERVING:

196 Calories

6 g Protein

7 g Total fat

1 g Saturated fat

0 g Monounsaturated fat

30 g Carbohydrates

5 g Fiber

2 g Sugar

54 mg Calcium

4 mg Iron

193 mg Sodium

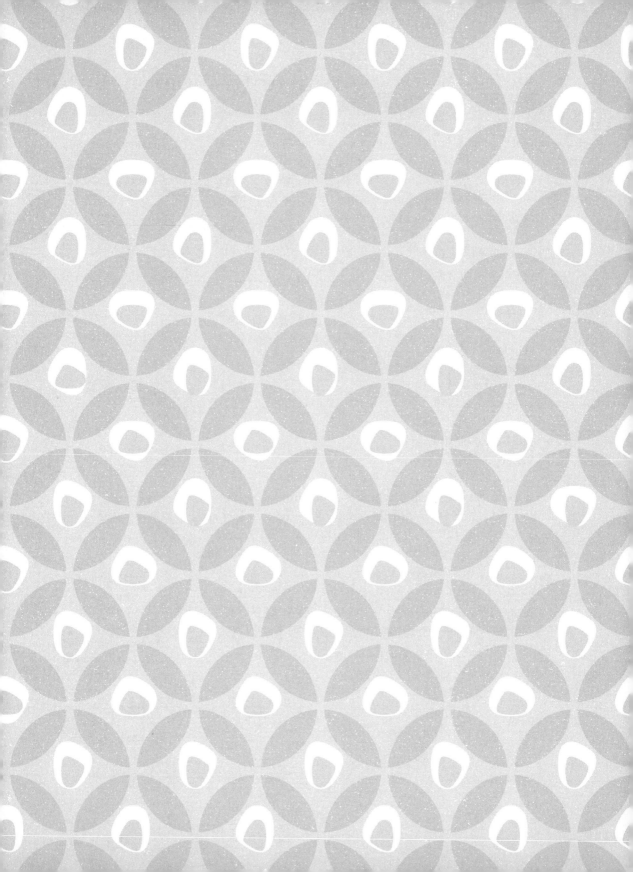

Soup's On!

IN GEORGIA THE mercury in the thermometer can reach up to 100 degrees or more in the summer. Add on a thick layer of humidity and you feel like you're in a constant outdoor sauna all day and all night. Even in this sweltering heat I find myself warming up a big bowl of soup and ladeling it into a thermos on my way to school or work at least twice a week. It seems that no matter the season and no matter what kind of soup it is, that warm bowl of goodness always falls under the heading of comfort food for me. Not only that, but soups are incredibly filling and can easily be eaten as a stand-alone meal or with a piece of crusty bread and a small salad.

Vegetable Noodle Soup

MAKES 4 SERVINGS

Try this on a cold winter day. I guarantee it's better than any chicken noodle soup you've ever had.

1 tablespoon extra virgin olive oil

1 cup diced celery

1 cup peeled and diced carrot

½ cup peeled and diced parsnip

½ cup diced white or yellow onion

5 cups vegetable stock

1 teaspoon dried thyme

4 ounces pasta, any shape

Warm the oil in a medium stockpot over medium-high heat. Add the celery, carrot, parsnip, and onion and cook, stirring frequently, for 2 minutes. Add the stock and thyme and bring to a boil. Add the pasta and cook for 15 to 17 minutes.

PER SERVING:

199 Calories

5 g Protein

5 g Total fat

1 g Saturated fat

0 g Monounsaturated fat

34 g Carbohydrates

3 g Fiber

6 g Sugar

48 mg Calcium

1 mg Iron

788 mg Sodium

Minestrone Soup

Not every soup falls neatly into the comfort food category, but Minestrone Soup fits the definition perfectly. It just makes you feel warm, comfy, and at home. I remember going out to lunch many a weekday afternoon with my old college roommate and eating minestrone soup and a salad while sipping sangria. This hodge-podge of fresh vegetables, beans, and pasta makes one of the most filling soups you will ever encounter.

2 tablespoons extra virgin olive oil

1 cup diced onion

1 small zucchini, diced

1 medium carrot, peeled and diced

1 celery stalk, diced

4 garlic cloves, minced

7 cups vegetable stock

One 14-ounce can petite diced tomatoes, drained

3 cups cooked kidney beans

3 cups cooked chickpeas

½ cup fresh or frozen green beans, cut into 1- to 2-inch pieces

1 teaspoon dried parsley

1 teaspoon dried oregano

½ teaspoon ground white pepper

½ teaspoon dried basil

½ teaspoon dried marjoram

½ teaspoon dried thyme

½ cup small shaped pasta, uncooked

4 cups fresh baby spinach

Warm the oil in a Dutch oven or large stockpot over medium heat. Add the onion, zucchini, carrot, celery, and garlic and cook until the onion begins to soften, about 5 minutes. Add the stock, tomatoes, kidney beans, chickpeas, green beans, parsley, oregano, white pepper, basil, marjoram, and thyme. Bring to a boil then reduce the heat, cover, and simmer for 15 minutes.

Add the pasta and cook, uncovered, for an additional 15 minutes. Stir in the baby spinach and cook until wilted.

MAKES 8 SERVINGS

PER SERVING:

264 Calories

15 g Protein

5 g Total fat

1 g Saturated fat

0 g Monounsaturated fat

43 g Carbohydrates

13 g Fiber

7 g Sugar

211 mg Calcium

5 mg Iron

715 mg Sodium

Sweet Pea Soup

MAKES 6 SERVINGS

This light, fragrant, and sweet soup is a great start to any meal. At only 98 calories it offers a whole lot more nutritional bang for your calorie buck than starting off your meal with bread and margarine. And if you have guests, this light soup will make you seem super fancy for serving a multiple-course dinner.

1 tablespoon Earth Balance margarine

1 bunch of scallions, sliced

2½ cups fresh or thawed sweet peas

¼ cup chopped fresh parsley

1 tablespoon sugar

¼ teaspoon fine sea salt

4 cups vegetable stock

1 tablespoon cornstarch

¼ cup water

Freshly ground black pepper to taste

Melt the margarine in a medium stockpot over medium heat then add the scallions and cook until soft and bright green, about 1 minute. Add the peas, parsley, sugar, salt, and stock and bring to a boil. Whisk together cornstarch and water in a small bowl and add to the pea mixture. Reduce the heat and simmer for about 5 minutes until thickened. Remove the pot from the heat and, in two batches, puree the soup in a blender. Season with black pepper to taste. Return the pureed soup to the stockpot and warm through if needed.

PER SERVING:

98 Calories

4 g Protein

2 g Total fat

1 g Saturated fat

0 g Monounsaturated fat

16 g Carbohydrates

4 g Fiber

4 g Sugar

32 mg Calcium

1 mg Iron

705 mg Sodium

Orange Cauliflower Soup

Orange cauliflower doesn't have a distinctly different taste than more common white cauliflower, it's true. However, we don't eat just with our mouths and taste buds; we also eat with our eyes. And a big, steaming bowl of creamy orange soup is so much more inviting than a bowl of stark white soup. For the eye appeal alone, it's worth searching for orange or even purple cauliflower to puree into this soup. If you absolutely can't find orange cauliflower, try this with white—it will still taste great.

MAKES 4 SERVINGS

1 head orange cauliflower (about 2½ pounds)

1 red potato, scrubbed and chopped

1½ cups vegetable stock

1½ cups water

1 teaspoon fine sea salt

Freshly ground black pepper to taste

Put the cauliflower, potato, stock, and water into a large saucepan and bring to a boil. Reduce the heat, cover, and simmer for 10 minutes or until the vegetables are tender. Transfer the cauliflower mixture to a blender then add the salt and black pepper and blend until smooth. Return to the saucepan and warm through if needed.

PER SERVING:

137 Calories

7 g Protein

1 g Total fat

0 g Saturated fat

0 g Monounsaturated fat

27 g Carbohydrates

9 g Fiber

6 g Sugar

57 mg Calcium

2 mg Iron

846 mg Sodium

Chipotle Butternut Squash Bisque

MAKES 6 SERVINGS

When autumn hits and butternut squash comes into season, I literally buy crates of them and start making soups and purees to preserve their flavor for year-round use. I typically make around four batches of Chipotle Butternut Squash Bisque to freeze and last me through the year. At only 182 calories per generous serving, it tastes much more indulgent than it actually is. If you plan on making the Toasted Butternut Squash Seeds, start them when the squash comes out of the oven so they can be baking while you work on the soup.

BISQUE

- 1 medium butternut squash (about 3 pounds)
- 2 tablespoons plus 1 teaspoon canola oil
- 1 cup diced onion
- 1 celery stalk, diced
- 1 medium carrot, peeled and diced
- 2 garlic cloves, minced
- 6 cups vegetable stock
- 1 chipotle pepper in adobo sauce

TOASTED BUTTERNUT SQUASH SEEDS

- Seeds from 1 medium butternut squash
- 1 teaspoon light brown sugar
- 1 teaspoon extra virgin olive oil

To make the bisque:

Preheat the oven to 400°F and line a baking sheet with nonstick foil or parchment paper.

Cut the squash in half and scoop out the seeds and membranes. Put the seeds and membranes into a colander and set aside.

Spread 1 teaspoon of the oil evenly over the cut sides of the butternut squash. Place the squash cut side down on the prepared baking sheet and roast for 45 minutes or until tender.

Warm the remaining 2 tablespoons oil in a medium stockpot over medium heat. Add the onion, celery, and carrot and sauté

PER SERVING
(WITHOUT SQUASH SEEDS):

182 Calories
3 g Protein
6 g Total fat
0 g Saturated fat
0 g Monounsaturated fat
34 g Carbohydrates
5 g Fiber
9 g Sugar
124 mg Calcium
2 mg Iron
575 mg Sodium

PER SERVING
(WITH SQUASH SEEDS):

239 Cal
5 g Protein
8 g Total Fat
1 g Saturated Fat
4 g Monounsaturated Fat
40 g Carbohydrates
5 g Fiber
10 g Sugar
130 mg Calcium
2 mg Iron
578 mg Sodium

---

until the carrots are bright orange and tender, about 10 minutes. Add the garlic and sauté for an additional minute then add the vegetable stock. Scoop out the flesh of the roasted squash and add to the stockpot, stirring to combine. Bring to a boil then reduce the heat, cover, and simmer for 30 minutes.

Remove the pot from the heat and, in two batches, puree the soup in a blender, adding the chipotle pepper to one of the batches. Return to the stockpot and warm through. Ladle into serving bowls and top with Toasted Butternut Squash Seeds, if desired.

To make the Toasted Butternut Squash Seeds:

Preheat the oven or toaster oven to 300°F and line another baking sheet with parchment paper. Separate the squash membranes in the colander from the seeds and discard the membranes. Run the seeds under cold water and drain, then transfer to a small bowl. Add the brown sugar and olive oil and toss together, then spread in a single layer on the prepared baking sheet. Bake until toasted, about 30 minutes.

Yellow Split Pea Soup

This might, quite frankly, be the best soup I have ever made. Hands down. It has everything you'd ever want from a soup: it's filling, it's sweet yet savory, it's ridiculously easy to throw together, and it freezes like a champ. All that with just a little over 200 calories.

4 bay leaves

7 cups vegetable stock

1 medium carrot, peeled and diced

1 teaspoon celery salt

1 pound dried yellow split peas

½ medium onion, diced

1 teaspoon sugar

½ teaspoon hickory liquid smoke

Combine all the ingredients in a medium stockpot and bring to a boil. Reduce the heat, cover, and cook until the peas are soft, about 40 to 45 minutes. Remove the bay leaves before serving.

PER SERVING:
214 Calories
14 g Protein
1 g Total fat
0 g Saturated fat
0 g Monounsaturated fat
39 g Carbohydrates
15 g Fiber
7 g Sugar
38 mg Calcium
3 mg Iron
499 mg Sodium

Black-Eyed Pea Soup

MAKES 4 SERVINGS

You have a couple options when it comes to the butternut squash puree you use for this soup. If butternut squash are in season, I recommend roasting a fresh squash and pureeing the flesh, following the method I use in Chipotle Butternut Squash Bisque (page 146). However, if time or season are not on your side, you can buy canned butternut squash or thaw some frozen butternut squash and puree that.

1 cup butternut squash puree

4 cups vegetable stock

¼ teaspoon cayenne

2 teaspoons agave nectar or pure maple syrup

3 cups cooked black-eyed peas

½ cup loosely packed cilantro, chopped or torn by hand

Combine the pureed butternut squash, vegetable stock, and cayenne in a medium stockpot or Dutch oven. Bring to a low boil over medium heat. Add the agave nectar and black-eyed peas. Bring the soup back to a boil, then reduce the heat and simmer, uncovered, for 5 minutes. Stir in the cilantro and serve.

PER SERVING:

216 Calories

11 g Protein

1 g Total fat

0 g Saturated fat

0 g Monounsaturated fat

42 g Carbohydrates

8 g Fiber

11 g Sugar

54 mg Calcium

3 mg Iron

562 mg Sodium

Refried Bean Soup

It simply isn't fair to relegate refried beans to bean burritos and the sides of plates of Mexican food. They're more than just a little something on the side of your plate; they make an incredibly yummy soup with the help of a few good ole-fashioned kitchen standbys like corn, black beans, and tomatoes. And at 273 calories a bowl, it's hard to resist.

1 recipe Refried Beans (page 112)

2 cups fresh corn

1½ cups cooked black beans

2 cups vegetable stock

One 14.5-ounce can petite diced tomatoes

½ cup water

One 4-ounce can mild diced green chiles

⅛ teaspoon ground cumin

Combine all the ingredients in a medium saucepan and bring to a boil. Reduce the heat and simmer, uncovered, for 10 minutes.

PER SERVING:

273 Calories

13 g Protein

7 g Total fat

1 g Saturated fat

0 g Monounsaturated fat

44 g Carbohydrates

11 g Fiber

4 g Sugar

76 mg Calcium

4 mg Iron

713 mg Sodium

Creamy Black Bean Soup

Sixty minutes of simmering time might not exactly go along with the "quick" in Quick and Easy Low-Cal Vegan Comfort Food, *but this soup is easy to make and so warm, creamy, and comforting. I usually put this soup on the back burner while I'm working on other recipes and the cooking time just flies by.*

1 tablespoon canola oil

¾ cup diced white onion

1 large carrot, diced

½ cup diced bell pepper of any color

4 garlic cloves, minced

6 cups cooked black beans

4 cups vegetable stock

2 tablespoons apple cider vinegar

1 tablespoon chili powder

½ teaspoon cayenne

½ teaspoon ground cumin

½ teaspoon fine sea salt

½ teaspoon hickory liquid smoke

Warm the oil in a medium stockpot over medium-low heat. Add the onion, carrot, bell pepper, and garlic and cook, stirring often, for 15 minutes or until the carrots are just barely tender. (Keep the heat low enough that the veggies don't brown and the garlic doesn't burn and turn bitter.)

Put 3 cups of the beans into a food processor with 1 cup of the vegetable stock. Process on high speed until smooth. When the vegetables are ready, add the pureed beans, the remaining 3 cups whole beans, and the remaining 3 cups vegetable stock to the pot, along with the vinegar, chili powder, cayenne, cumin, salt, and liquid smoke. Bring to a boil, then reduce the heat and simmer, uncovered, for 50 to 60 minutes until the soup has thickened and all the ingredients are tender.

PER SERVING:

212 Calories

12 g Protein

3 g Total fat

0 g Saturated fat

1 g Monounsaturated fat

37 g Carbohydrates

12 g Fiber

3 g Sugar

50 mg Calcium

3 mg Iron

443 mg Sodium

Meatball Soup 📷

MAKES 6 SERVINGS

Meatball soup gives you a whole lot of bang for your nutritional buck. It is less than 250 calories a serving, and it has 17 grams of protein, 9 grams of fiber, 6 grams of iron, and almost as much calcium as a glass of milk! It's hard to imagine you can fit all that goodness into one hearty bowl of soup but in the land of Quick and Easy Low-Cal Vegan Comfort Food *anything is possible.*

MEATBALLS

1 cup dark vegetable stock

1 teaspoon hickory liquid smoke

1 teaspoon vegan Worcestershire sauce

1 cup textured vegetable protein (TVP)

¾ cup unseasoned bread crumbs

1 tablespoon vital wheat gluten

2 tablespoons minced fresh parsley

2 garlic cloves, minced

¼ cup plus 3 tablespoons ketchup

¼ teaspoon fine sea salt

¼ teaspoon ground black pepper

SOUP

1 tablespoon extra virgin olive oil

½ cup diced onion

1 celery rib, chopped

2 garlic cloves, chopped

One 14.5-ounce can petite diced tomatoes, with their juices

2 tablespoons tomato paste

3½ cups vegetable stock

1½ cups water

¼ teaspoon Italian seasoning

½ cup small shaped pasta

3 cups baby spinach leaves

2 tablespoons chopped fresh basil

PER SERVING:

231 Calories
17 g Protein
4 g Total fat
1 g Saturated fat
2 g Monounsaturated fat
35 g Carbohydrates
9 g Fiber
12 g Sugar
280 mg Calcium
6 mg Iron
1063 mg Sodium

To make the meatballs:

Bring the stock, liquid smoke, and Worcestershire sauce to a boil in a small pot. Remove from the heat, add the TVP, and let sit for 5 minutes.

Using your hands, combine the reconstituted TVP, bread crumbs, vital wheat gluten, parsley, garlic, ketchup, salt, and black pepper in a medium bowl. Form balls about the size of a rounded tablespoon and place them on a large plate or baking dish. Refrigerate for about an hour.

Preheat the oven to 350°F and line a baking sheet with parchment paper.

Arrange the meatballs on the baking sheet in a single layer and spray with nonstick cooking spray. Bake for 10 minutes then flip the meatballs over and spray with nonstick cooking spray. Bake until browned and firm, another 10 to 15 minutes.

To make the soup:

Warm the oil in a medium stockpot over medium heat. Add the onion and celery and cook until soft, 3 to 4 minutes. Add the garlic and cook for another minute. Add the tomatoes, tomato paste, stock, water, and Italian seasoning, and stir to combine. Bring to a boil then reduce the heat and simmer, uncovered, for 15 minutes.

Add the pasta and cook for an additional 15 minutes or until the pasta is cooked through. Stir in the spinach, basil, and cooked meatballs and cook until the spinach is wilted.

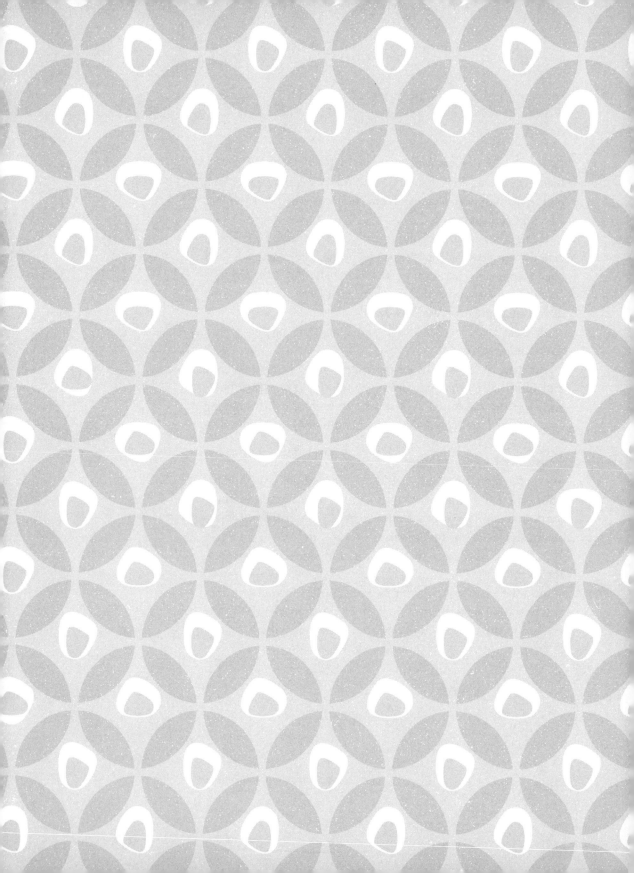

The Main Event

THIS IS IT—THE main event, the culinary part of the day you are looking most forward to. I hesitate to label this section as lunch or dinner because the two are completely interchangeable in my life. Are you dipping your toe into veganism and trying to figure out what to eat for dinner? Well, this section is for you! Are you a seasoned vegan just trying to spice up your lunch? Well, this section is for you, too! No matter who you are or what you're looking for this section is built to make your life easier, your taste buds happy, and your stomach full, all for less than 350 calories.

White Lasagna

MAKES 10 SERVINGS

This lasagna is all ooey, gooey, creamy deliciousness, and there isn't a casserole dish known to man that can contain it all. You'll need to dig out your deepest, largest baking dish for this one. Also, it expands as it cooks, so it can create quite a mess of your oven if you're not careful. I recommend placing a foil-lined baking sheet under the casserole dish to catch any bits of goo that try to escape.

One 14-ounce package extra-firm tofu

1 tablespoon Italian seasoning

1 tablespoon fresh lemon juice

1 teaspoon fine sea salt

¼ cup extra virgin olive oil

3 garlic cloves, minced

½ cup unbleached all-purpose flour

6 cups plain soy milk

One 18-ounce bag baby spinach

One 10-ounce package frozen peas

5 medium carrots, peeled, thinly sliced, and steamed until tender

2 cups broccoli florets, chopped and steamed

¼ teaspoon freshly ground black pepper

9 ounces lasagna noodles, uncooked

4 cups vegan mozzarella cheese, shredded

PER SERVING:

334 Calories

17 g Protein

11 g Total fat

1 g Saturated fat

42 g Carbohydrates

7 g Fiber

6 g Sugar

339 mg Calcium

4 mg Iron

480 mg Sodium

Preheat the oven to 425°F. Lightly spray a 9 x 13-inch casserole dish with nonstick cooking spray.

Mash the tofu with the Italian seasoning, lemon juice, and ½ teaspoon of the salt. Stir until the tofu is well coated and set aside.

Warm the oil in a large saucepan over medium heat. Add the garlic and cook, stirring constantly, for 1 minute. Whisk in the flour and continue to whisk until incorporated into the oil, about another minute. Slowly whisk in the milk. Bring to a low boil then reduce the heat and simmer, stirring occasionally, until sauce begins to thicken, about 5 minutes. Add the spinach, peas, carrots, broccoli, black pepper, and the remaining

½ teaspoon salt. Continue to stir and cook until spinach wilts. Remove from the heat.

Spread enough vegetable sauce in the casserole dish to cover the bottom. Add 1 layer of lasagna noodles. Pour half the remaining vegetable sauce over the noodles, then cover with half the mashed tofu and half the vegan mozzarella cheese. Add a second layer of noodles and repeat with the remaining ingredients. Cover with nonstick aluminum foil.

Bake for 45 minutes. Remove the foil and bake for an additional 15 minutes. If all the cheese hasn't melted, put lasagna under the broiler until the cheese is melted and bubbling. Allow to cool slightly before serving—the lasagna will be hot!

Fettuccine Slim-Fredo

MAKES 8 SERVINGS

The two recipes from my first book, Quick and Easy Vegan Comfort Food, *that I get the most e-mails about are Mac and Cheeze and Fettuccine Alfredo Two Ways. Admittedly, the key ingredient that makes my Fettuccine Alfredo so delicious is lots and lots of oil. Well, lots and lots of oil doesn't fit the low-cal description, so I modified the recipe to make it more waistline friendly without sacrificing the taste. At 345 calories you have a complete meal, with a generous portion of pasta, creamy Alfredo sauce, and fresh crisp broccoli.*

1 pound dry fettuccine pasta

Two 12-ounce packages soft silken tofu

½ cup canola oil

¼ cup unsweetened plain soy milk

1 teaspoon onion powder

½ cup nutritional yeast

2 teaspoons fine sea salt

3 garlic cloves, chopped

Freshly ground black pepper to taste

1 head broccoli, cut into florets and steamed

Cook the pasta according to the directions on the package. While the pasta is cooking, put the tofu, oil, milk, onion powder, nutritional yeast, salt, garlic, and black pepper into a blender and blend until smooth. Drain the pasta and briefly set aside. Pour the tofu mixture into the pot the pasta cooked in and warm over medium heat until the sauce begins to bubble. Add the cooked pasta and broccoli to the sauce and toss to coat.

PER SERVING:

345 Calories

16 g Protein

18 g Total fat

2 g Saturated fat

0 g Monounsaturated fat

40 g Carbohydrates

3 g Fiber

2 g Sugar

73 mg Calcium

3 mg Iron

63 mg Sodium

Open-Faced Black Bean Burger with Spiced Ketchup 📷

MAKES 6 BURGERS

With the help of a food processor, making black bean burgers is quick and easy. I don't know how my kitchen would function without one! If you don't yet have a food processor, it's a worthwhile investment, but you can use a blender for this recipe in the meantime. These burgers can be made ahead and kept in the refrigerator for up to 3 days before cooking.

½ cup diced white or yellow onion

½ cup diced red bell pepper

3 cups cooked black beans

¾ cup cooked brown rice

½ teaspoon fine sea salt

1 teaspoon ground cumin

¼ cup plain bread crumbs

3 hamburger buns, cut in half

¼ cup plus 2 tablespoons Spiced Ketchup (page 232)

1 cup fresh baby spinach

Put the onions, bell pepper, beans, rice, salt, and cumin into a food processor and process until most of the black beans are mashed but some small pieces of beans are still visible. Transfer the bean mixture to a large bowl and fold in the bread crumbs.

Form the mixture into 6 balls of about ½ cup each then flatten into patties. Refrigerate for at least 15 minutes and up to 3 days.

Preheat the oven to 350°F and line a baking sheet with non-stick aluminum foil or parchment paper.

Arrange the patties on the prepared baking sheet and spray with nonstick cooking spray. Bake for 15 minutes, then turn patties over and spray again with nonstick cooking spray. Bake for an additional 15 minutes. Place each patty on a bun half and top with Spiced Ketchup and spinach.

PER BURGER:

195 Calories

11 g Protein

1 g Total fat

0 g Saturated fat

0 g Monounsaturated fat

37 g Carbohydrates

10 g Fiber

5 g Sugar

92 mg Calcium

3 mg Iron

430 mg Sodium

Carolina BBQ Sammich

MAKES 4 SANDWICHES

These can be served two ways: open-faced or as a traditional two-bun sammy. For the open-faced option you'll only need 2 buns; you'll need 4 to go for the full sammy.

1 tablespoon canola oil

½ medium red bell pepper, thinly sliced

One 8-ounce package tempeh, any variety, thinly sliced

1 cup Sweet Caroline BBQ Sauce (page 233)

2 or 4 hamburger buns, toasted

**PER SANDWICH
(TRADITIONAL STYLE):**
334 Calories
16 g Protein
10 g Total fat
1 g Saturated fat
2 g Monounsaturated fat
58 g Carbohydrates
8 g Fiber
23 g Sugar
155 mg Calcium
3 mg Iron
717 mg Sodium

**PER SANDWICH
(OPEN-FACED):**
284 Calories
14 g Protein
9 g Total fat
1 g Saturated fat
2 g Monounsaturated fat
44 g Carbohydrates
8 g Fiber
20 g Sugar
125 mg Calcium
2 mg Iron
582 mg Sodium

Warm the oil in a large skillet over medium heat. Add the bell pepper and cook for 1 minute. Add the tempeh and cook, gently stirring, for 4 to 5 minutes until the tempeh is warmed through. Stir in the Sweet Caroline BBQ Sauce and cook until warmed. Serve on the toasted buns.

Ballpark Hot Dogs

For centuries and centuries, people have wondered why hot dogs come in a pack of six but hot dog buns come in a pack of eight—well, perhaps not centuries, but it sure does feel like it! This recipe for big, juicy ballpark hot dogs makes exactly eight hot dogs to solve this ancient problem once and for all.

1 tablespoon Bragg Liquid Aminos

1 tablespoon extra virgin olive oil

1½ tablespoons ketchup

1 garlic clove, chopped

¼ cup diced onion

2 teaspoons light brown sugar

¾ cup plus 2 tablespoons water

1 cup vital wheat gluten

¾ cup soy flour

¼ cup nutritional yeast

2½ teaspoons smoked paprika

½ teaspoon ground cumin

½ teaspoon ground allspice

¼ teaspoon ground white pepper

1 teaspoon ground coriander

8 reduced-calorie hot dog buns, about 80 calories per bun

Put the liquid aminos, oil, ketchup, garlic, onion, and brown sugar into a food processor and process until smooth. Slowly pour in water, pulsing to combine. Set aside.

Combine the gluten, soy flour, nutritional yeast, paprika, cumin, allspice, white pepper, and coriander in a small bowl. Add the liquid aminos mixture to the gluten mixture and mix well, forming a soft wet dough.

Divide the dough into 8 balls then roll each into a 6-inch log. Place each log onto a separate piece of aluminum foil and wrap tightly. (If you don't wrap the hot dogs tightly enough in the foil, they will burst out during cooking.) Twist the ends of the foil to seal. Steam for 30 minutes.

Remove the hot dogs from the foil then place each in a bun and top with your favorite toppings.

MAKE 8 HOT DOGS

PER HOT DOG (WITHOUT BUN):

119 Calories

18 g Protein

2 g Total fat

0 g Saturated fat

0 g Monounsaturated fat

11 g Carbohydrates

3 g Fiber

4 g Sugar

53 mg Calcium

2 mg Iron

161 mg Sodium

PER HOT DOG (WITH REDUCED-CALORIE BUN):

199 Calories

22 g Protein

3 g Total fat

0 g Saturated fat

0 g Monounsaturated fat

26 g Carbohydrates

9 g Fiber

6 g Sugar

153 mg Calcium

4 mg Iron

321 mg Sodium

Corn Dogs 📷

My handy bread machine lets me throw all the ingredients for corn dog dough into it, set it on the dough cycle, and get to work making my Ballpark Hot Dogs. By the time the dough is finished, the hot dogs are ready. Then it's time to assemble the corn dogs and get the mustard ready for dipping. Don't worry—if you don't have a bread machine, you can still make these corn dogs!

1 cup plain almond milk

2¼ teaspoons active dry yeast or bread machine yeast

2 tablespoons canola oil

2 tablespoons light brown sugar

1 cup corn flour

1¼ cup bread flour

1 teaspoon fine sea salt

½ teaspoon baking soda

1 recipe Ballpark Hot Dogs (page 161)

To make in a bread machine:

Put the milk, yeast, oil, sugar, corn flour, bread flour, salt, and baking soda into a bread machine according to the manufacturer's directions and choose the dough cycle (use the 1-pound setting).

Preheat the oven to 450°F and line a baking sheet with parchment paper.

When the dough is finished, turn out onto a lightly floured surface and divide into 8 pieces. Roll each piece into a 10- to 12-inch rope. Wrap each rope of dough around a hot dog and press the edges together to seal. Place on the prepared baking sheet.

Spray the corn dogs lightly with nonstick cooking spray and bake for 15 minutes or until golden.

To make on the stove:

Warm the milk in a small saucepan then transfer to a medium bowl. Sprinkle in the yeast and let sit for 2 minutes. Stir in the oil, brown sugar, corn flour, bread flour, salt, and baking soda and mix to form a soft, sticky dough.

PER CORN DOG:

297 Calories

22 g Protein

7 g Total fat

1 g Saturated fat

0 g Monounsaturated fat

42 g Carbohydrates

6 g Fiber

7 g Sugar

60 mg Calcium

4 mg Iron

537 mg Sodium

Turn the dough out onto a lightly floured surface and knead, adding more flour if needed, until smooth but still a little sticky. Shape the dough into a ball and place in a lightly oiled bowl. Cover with plastic wrap and set in a warm place to rise until doubled in size, about an hour.

Preheat the oven to 450°F and line a baking sheet with parchment paper. Turn the dough out onto a lightly floured surface and divide into 8 pieces. Roll each piece into a 10- to 12-inch rope. Wrap each rope of dough around a hot dog and press the edges together to seal. Place on the prepared baking sheet.

Spray the corn dogs lightly with nonstick cooking spray and bake for 15 minutes or until golden.

Chili Dogs

MAKES 8 CHILI DOGS

Chili was made for hot dogs—or is it that chili was made for Chili Cheese Fries (page 165)? I can never decide. But whether you prefer your chili on fries or dogs, I've got you covered.

1 recipe Ballpark Hot Dogs (page 161)
½ recipe for Ole-Fashioned Chili Beans (page 169)
8 reduced-calorie hot dog buns

PER CHILI DOG:
273 Calories
28 g Protein
4 g Total fat
0 g Saturated fat
0 g Monounsaturated fat
40 g Carbohydrates
13 g Fiber
9 g Sugar
188 mg Calcium
5 mg Iron
666 mg Sodium

Place each Ballpark Hot Dog into a bun and top with a generous serving of Ole-Fashioned Chili Beans.

Chili Cheese Dogs

**PER
CHILI CHEESE DOG:**
307 Calories
28 g Protein
6 g Total fat
0 g Saturated fat
0 g Monounsaturated fat
44 g Carbohydrates
14 g Fiber
9 g Sugar
193 mg Calcium
6 mg Iron
781 mg Sodium

1 recipe Chili Dogs
½ recipe Classic Cheese Sauce (page 237)

Spoon Classic Cheese Sauce over the chili beans, distributing evenly among the 8 chili dogs.

Chili Cheese Fries 📷

Make no mistake about it, chili cheese fries are a full meal. They've got everything you need: veggies, protein, starch, fruit . . . well, maybe not fruit, though beans have been referred to as "the magical fruit." Either way, all you need are these Chili Cheese Fries and a small salad and you're set for lunch or dinner.

MAKES 6 SERVINGS

3 large russet potatoes, scrubbed and cut into ¼- to ½-inch-thick strips

1½ tablespoons canola oil

½ teaspoon fine sea salt

¼ teaspoon paprika

1 recipe Classic Cheese Sauce (page 237)

½ recipe Ole-Fashioned Chili Beans (page 169)

Preheat the oven to 450°F and line a baking sheet with nonstick foil or parchment paper.

Toss the potatoes with oil then salt and paprika in a large bowl. Arrange on the baking sheet in a single layer. Bake for 30 minutes or until golden brown and crispy. Divide the fries among serving plates and top with cheese sauce and chili beans.

PER SERVING:

286 Calories

11 g Protein

8 g Total fat

0 g Saturated fat

0 g Monounsaturated fat

44 g Carbohydrates

9 g Fiber

4 g Sugar

72 mg Calcium

4 mg Iron

967 mg Sodium

Poke and Beans

I stopped eating pork when I was barely old enough to spell my own name, so I don't remember much about it but I do still distinctly remember the taste of pork and beans. Actually, as a child, I would always eat around the pork and dive straight for the beans and that sweet syrupy sauce they swam in. My version of the canned classic mixes it up a little with kidney beans but keeps it simple with bell pepper, onion, brown sugar, maple syrup, and ketchup.

1 tablespoon canola oil

4 Ballpark Hot Dogs (page 161) or commercial vegan hot dogs, sliced

1 cup diced red bell pepper

½ cup diced white onion

½ cup light brown sugar

¼ cup pure maple syrup

1 cup ketchup

1 teaspoon garlic powder

2 cups water

4 cups cooked navy beans

2 cups cooked kidney beans

Warm the oil in a large saucepan over medium heat. Add the hot dogs, bell pepper, and onion and cook for 3 minutes. Add the brown sugar, maple syrup, ketchup, and garlic powder and bring to a low boil. Add the water, navy beans, and kidney beans and bring back to a boil. Reduce the heat and simmer, uncovered, for 20 minutes or until thickened.

PER SERVING:

338 Calories

17 g Protein

3 g Total fat

0 g Saturated fat

0 g Monounsaturated fat

64 g Carbohydrates

10 g Fiber

27 g Sugar

110 mg Calcium

4 mg Iron

499 mg Sodium

Backyard Beans

These beans are a potluck favorite. They're a little sweet, a little savory, and packed full of fiber and protein thanks to 5 types of dry beans, a little TVP, and some green beans—just to make sure you eat your vegetables!

MAKES 10 SERVINGS

3 cups vegetable stock

1 teaspoon vegan Worcestershire sauce

1 teaspoon hickory liquid smoke

1 cup textured vegetable protein (TVP)

1 tablespoon canola oil

½ medium onion, diced

4 garlic cloves, minced

1½ cups cooked kidney beans

1½ cups cooked navy beans

1½ cups cooked black beans

1½ cups cooked pinto beans

½ teaspoon red pepper flakes

1 cup Sweet Caroline BBQ Sauce (page 233)

¼ cup light brown sugar

One 28-ounce can tomato sauce

One 12-ounce package frozen cut green beans

One 10-ounce package frozen lima beans

Put 1 cup of the vegetable stock and the Worcestershire sauce and liquid smoke into a small saucepan and bring to a low boil. Stir in the TVP and let sit for 5 minutes. Set aside.

Warm the oil in a Dutch oven or large saucepan over medium heat. Add the onion and cook until softened, about 2 minutes. Add the garlic and cook until fragrant, about 30 seconds. Stir in the kidney beans, navy beans, black beans, pinto beans, red pepper flakes, barbecue sauce, brown sugar, and tomato sauce and bring to a boil. Reduce the heat, cover, and simmer for 30 minutes. Add the green beans and lima beans and cook for an additional 15 minutes.

PER SERVING:

307 Calories

17 g Protein

3 g Total fat

0 g Saturated fat

0 g Monounsaturated fat

56 g Carbohydrates

13 g Fiber

18 g Sugar

125 mg Calcium

5 mg Iron

852 mg Sodium

Pinto Beans in Ancho Chile Sauce

MAKES 4 SERVINGS

These beans are endlessly versatile. They can be smashed into Refried Beans (page 112), used as a filling for tacos or burritos or as a topping for nachos, or simply served over a bed of rice with a side of veggies.

1 tablespoon canola oil

2 to 3 tablespoons Ancho Chile Sauce (page 235)

3½ cups cooked pinto beans

2 bay leaves

3 cups vegetable stock

Warm the oil in a medium saucepan then add the chile sauce and cook for 1 minute. Add the beans, bay leaves, and stock and bring to a boil. Reduce the heat and simmer, uncovered, for 10 minutes. Discard the bay leaves before serving.

PER SERVING:

259 Calories

14 g Protein

5 g Total fat

0 g Saturated fat

0 g Monounsaturated fat

41 g Carbohydrates

13 g Fiber

2 g Sugar

69 mg Calcium

4 mg Iron

489 mg Sodium

Ole-Fashioned Chili Beans

Chili is one of those dishes that seems like it should be full of calories but is so light it ought to be a crime. At 154 calories for each big, steaming bowl of Ole-Fashioned Chili Beans, you'll have more than enough calories to spare for a slice of Masa Cornbread (page 85), some steamed veggies on the side, and even dessert.

MAKES 6 SERVINGS

1½ cups cooked kidney beans

1½ cups cooked pinto beans

½ cup textured vegetable protein (TVP)

One 28-ounce can diced tomatoes, with juices

1 cup water

1 teaspoon ground cumin

1 teaspoon paprika

2 tablespoons chili powder

1 teaspoon dried oregano

½ teaspoon fine sea salt

¼ teaspoon freshly ground black pepper

1 teaspoon onion powder

1 teaspoon garlic powder

¼ teaspoon red pepper flakes

½ teaspoon ground allspice

To make on the stove:

Combine all the ingredients in a medium stockpot over medium-high heat and bring to a boil. Lower the heat and simmer, uncovered, for 15 minutes.

To make in a slow cooker:

Combine all the ingredients in the slow cooker and cook on the low setting for at least 4 hours, up to 8 hours.

PER SERVING:

154 Calories

9 g Protein

1 g Total fat

0 g Saturated fat

0 g Monounsaturated fat

29 g Carbohydrates

9 g Fiber

4 g Sugar

64 mg Calcium

3 mg Iron

235 mg Sodium

Cincinnati Chili

MAKES 10 SERVINGS

When I first heard of Cincinnati Chili, I couldn't imagine how spaghetti and chili could taste remotely good together. The whole concept was completely bizarre to me. But spaghetti isn't the only thing that makes Cincinnati Chili stand out. The mix of aromatic herbs and spices with just the right amount of chocolate undertone makes it a crowd pleaser, and kids love the combination of the two very kid-friendly foods.

1 tablespoon extra virgin olive oil

1 medium onion, diced

6 garlic cloves, minced

6 cups vegetable stock

1 teaspoon hickory liquid smoke

2 cups textured vegetable protein (TVP)

2 tablespoons unsweetened cocoa powder

1½ teaspoons ground allspice

1½ teaspoons ground cinnamon

½ teaspoon cayenne

¼ teaspoon ground cloves

⅓ cup tomato paste

1 tablespoon apple cider vinegar

1½ tablespoons chili powder

1 tablespoon dried oregano

1 tablespoon light brown sugar

1 tablespoon vegan Worcestershire sauce

3 cups cooked kidney beans

1 pound dry spaghetti

¼ cup chopped fresh parsley

PER SERVING:

241 Calories

16 g Protein

2 g Total fat

0 g Saturated fat

0 g Monounsaturated fat

39 g Carbohydrates

11 g Fiber

7 g Sugar

111 mg Calcium

5 mg Iron

455 mg Sodium

Warm the oil in a large deep skillet, like a braising skillet, over medium heat. Add the onion and sauté until soft, about 5 minutes. Add the garlic and cook until fragrant, about 1 minute. Add 2 cups of the stock and the liquid smoke and bring to a low boil. Reduce the heat, then stir in the TVP and allow to sit until it absorbs all the liquid, about 3 minutes. Increase the heat to medium and stir in the cocoa, allspice, cinnamon, cayenne, cloves, tomato paste, vinegar, chili powder, oregano, brown sugar, Worcestershire sauce, kidney beans, and remaining 4 cups stock. Bring to a boil then reduce the heat and simmer, uncovered and stirring often, until thickened, about 30 minutes.

While chili is simmering, cook the spaghetti according to the directions on the package.

Stir in 2 tablespoons parsley into the cooked chili. Divide the spaghetti among 10 bowls then top with chili. Garnish with the remaining 2 tablespoons parsley.

Black Bean Quesadillas with Roasted Tomatillo Salsa

MAKES 4 QUESADILLAS

The salsa is what makes these quesadillas special. As tempting as it is to pull out a jar of that store-bought stuff, nothing can compare to the taste of warm Roasted Tomatillo Salsa made with fresh, pure ingredients. And don't stop at using it on these quesadillas—make a double batch and try it on Baked Tortilla Chips (page 98) or Southwest Scramble (page 54), too!

ROASTED TOMATILLO SALSA (MAKES ¾ CUP)

1 head garlic, top cut off

1 tablespoon plus 1 teaspoon canola oil

¾ pounds tomatillos (about 8), husks discarded, rinsed, and cut in half

½ medium onion, cut into wedges

½ serrano chile pepper (see Cook's Tip)

¼ teaspoon fine sea salt

⅛ teaspoon ground black pepper

2 tablespoons vegetable stock

1 tablespoon minced fresh cilantro

QUESADILLAS

½ small onion, thinly sliced

½ medium bell pepper of any color, thinly sliced

1 cup cooked black beans

1 cup Chickpea Cheese (page 101)

4 large flour tortillas

PER QUESADILLA
(WITH SALSA):

348 Calories

11 g Protein

11 g Total fat

1 g Saturated fat

5 g Monounsaturated fat

52 g Carbohydrates

8 g Fiber

7 g Sugar

94 mg Calcium

4 mg Iron

569 mg Sodium

PER SERVING
OF SALSA ONLY
(2 TABLESPOONS):

57 Calories

1 g Protein

4 g Total fat

0 g Saturated fat

0 g Monounsaturated fat

6 g Carbohydrates

1 g Fiber

3 g Sugar

10 mg Calcium

0 mg Iron

111 mg Sodium

To make the salsa:

Preheat the oven to 350°F and line a baking sheet with nonstick foil or parchment paper.

Place the head of garlic on a small piece of foil and drizzle with 1 teaspoon of the oil. Wrap tightly and place on the prepared baking sheet. Place the tomatillos, onion, and chile pepper cut side up on the prepared baking sheet. Drizzle with remaining 1 tablespoon oil and sprinkle with the salt and pepper. Roast for 30 to 40 minutes until vegetables are soft.

Transfer the roasted vegetables to a food processor or blender. Squeeze the roasted garlic out of the skins and add to the vegetables. Add the stock and process until smooth. Transfer to a bowl. Stir in the cilantro and serve warm or cold.

To prepare the quesadillas:

Warm a large dry skillet or saucepan (preferably cast iron) over medium heat. Add the onion and bell pepper and sauté for 2 to 3 minutes until they begin to become translucent. Set aside.

Spoon ¼ cup of Chickpea Cheese into the center of each tortilla then spread evenly, leaving an inch around the edge.

Warm a separate large skillet over medium heat. Place 1 tortilla, cheese side up, onto the hot pan. Spoon ¼ cup black beans and ¼ of the onion mixture onto one side of the tortilla. Fold the tortilla in half. Cook until slightly crispy on the bottom, then flip and cook the other side until crispy and the cheese is melted. Repeat with the remaining tortillas and fillings. Cut each quesadilla in half and serve topped with 2 tablespoons of Roasted Tomatillo Salsa.

Cook's Tip: Wherever fresh chile peppers are called for, you can greatly reduce the amount of heat they contribute to your dish by removing and discarding their seeds and membranes. If you like it hot, go ahead and use them.

Plantain and Black Bean Tamales

MAKES 24 TAMALES

I adore tamales, but unfortunately they're not the least bit quick to make—at least, not all by yourself. Making tamales is a fun activity to do with the entire family, and—more to the point—a group of people spreading masa dough, filling tamales, and wrapping them up can accomplish in 10 minutes what would take one person 30.

24 corn husks

3¼ cups masa harina

2 teaspoons baking powder

½ teaspoon garlic powder

½ teaspoon fine sea salt

½ cup vegetable shortening

3 cups vegetable stock

2 large very ripe plantains

1 tablespoon canola oil

3¼ cups cooked black beans

3 tablespoons plus 1½ teaspoons Ancho Chile Sauce (page 235)

Submerge the corn husks in a large bowl of warm water to soften. Set aside.

Combine the masa harina, baking powder, garlic powder, and salt in a large bowl. Beat in the shortening with an electric mixer or large spoon. Add ½ cup of the stock and beat well. Continue to add ½ cup of stock at a time, beating well after each addition, until you have a consistency that you can spread with a knife.

Peel the plantains and cut diagonally into ½-inch-thick pieces. Warm the oil in a large skillet over medium heat and place half the plantains pieces in the skillet. Cook for 3 to 4 minutes on each side or until golden brown. Remove to a plate and repeat with the remaining plantain.

Combine the beans and chile sauce in a medium bowl.

PER TAMALE:

150 Calories

4 g Protein

6 g Total fat

1 g Saturated fat

2 g Monounsaturated fat

23 g Carbohydrates

4 g Fiber

3 g Sugar

51 mg Calcium

2 mg Iron

160 mg Sodium

To prepare the tamales:

Spread a layer of masa dough evenly in the middle third of each corn husk, leaving the sides and ends bare. (Use your hands to spread the masa if you need to.) Place one slice of cooked plantain and then 2 tablespoons of black bean mixture over the masa. Fold the sides of the husk over the masa so that they overlap each other completely, then fold the ends over in the same way to make a square packet. Make sure none of the filling leaks out. Place the tamale, seam side down, in a steamer. Repeat with remaining corn husks and fillings.

Steam the tamales for 40 to 45 minutes. They are cooked when the filling separates easily from the corn husk.

Wet Burritos

There's nothing particularly pretty about these burritos, but what they lack in beauty they make up for in yum.

1 cup vegetable stock

1½ teaspoons hickory liquid smoke

1 cup textured vegetable protein (TVP)

1 tablespoon canola oil

½ cup diced white or yellow onion

1 medium red bell pepper, diced

2 cloves garlic, minced

1 tablespoon water

2 tablespoons Taco Seasoning Mix (page 234)

3 cups Enchilada Sauce (page 236)

4 large flour tortillas

2 cups Refried Beans (page 112) or Refried Black Beans (page 113)

4 large leaves green leaf lettuce, shredded

3 scallions, chopped

Put the stock and liquid smoke into a small pot and bring to a boil. Remove from the heat then add the TVP and let sit for 5 minutes.

Warm the oil in a medium saucepan over medium-high heat. Add the onion and bell pepper and cook for 2 to 3 minutes until the onions are translucent and the bell peppers soften. Add the garlic and sauté for an additional minute. Add the rehydrated TVP, water, and the taco seasoning. Cook, stirring, until all the water has been absorbed and the taco seasoning is evenly distributed.

If Enchilada Sauce is not already warm, warm it in a small saucepan over medium heat.

Soften the tortillas in the microwave, about 10 seconds per tortilla.

Spoon the TVP mixture, refried beans, and lettuce onto the softened tortillas, distributing the fillings evenly. Roll up the burritos and place, seam side down, on serving plates. Cut in half then spoon warm Enchilada Sauce over each burrito and garnish with the chopped scallions.

PER BURRITO:

289 Calories

15 g Protein

7 g Total fat

1 g Saturated fat

4 g Monounsaturated fat

41 g Carbohydrates

10 g Fiber

6 g Sugar

138 mg Calcium

5 mg Iron

1451 mg Sodium

Pigeon Peas and Rice

Don't be scared off by the Scotch bonnet in this recipe: when you add the whole, intact pepper, you don't get the extreme heat a pepper of this caliber normally delivers. Instead, it subtly seasons the rice and peas, and the cooked pepper makes a beautiful garnish for the finished dish. If you're truly daring, you might even take a bite—although I'm not, and probably will never be, that brave.

MAKES 8 SERVINGS

1 tablespoon canola oil

½ medium onion, diced

4 garlic cloves, minced

2 cups uncooked brown rice

1 teaspoon grated fresh ginger

½ teaspoon fine sea salt

1 cup water

1½ cups vegetable stock

One 13- to 14-ounce can light coconut milk

One 15-ounce can pigeon peas, rinsed and drained

2 teaspoons dried thyme

1 bay leaf

1 Scotch bonnet pepper

Warm the oil in a large saucepan over medium heat. Add the onions and sauté for 4 to 5 minutes until translucent. Add the garlic and rice and cook for another 2 to 3 minutes, stirring often. Add the ginger, salt, water, stock, and coconut milk and stir well. Stir in the pigeon peas, thyme, bay leaf, and Scotch bonnet pepper and bring to a low boil. Reduce the heat, cover, and simmer until the rice is tender, about 30 minutes.

Remove the pan from the heat and allow to sit, covered, for an additional 5 minutes. Remove the bay leaf and Scotch bonnet pepper. Stir the peas and rice to evenly distribute the ingredients.

PER SERVING:

291 Calories

8 g Protein

6 g Total fat

3 g Saturated fat

0 g Monounsaturated fat

52 g Carbohydrates

6 g Fiber

1 g Sugar

33 mg Calcium

1 mg Iron

258 mg Sodium

Andouille Gumbo

MAKES 10 SERVINGS

Before penning Quick and Easy Vegan Celebrations *I had never eaten gumbo in my life. The mix of seafood and okra just seemed like the most unappealing thing in the world to me. While experimenting with gumbo recipes for* Vegan Celebrations, *I found myself making it nearly once a week for a six-month stretch! I now have at least a dozen gumbo recipes in my arsenal, and this is one of my favorites. It's hard to believe that a recipe that starts with a half cup of margarine could be considered low-calorie, but surprisingly, this gumbo is only 322 calories per serving, including the rice you serve it with.*

½ cup Earth Balance margarine

½ cup unbleached all-purpose flour

3 Andouille Sausage links (page 43), cut into ¼-inch-thick slices

¾ cup diced white or yellow onion

1 celery stalk, diced

½ medium red bell pepper, diced

½ medium green bell pepper, diced

2 small tomatoes, diced

2 tablespoons dried parsley

2 garlic cloves, minced

3 cups vegetable stock

2 bay leaves

1 teaspoon dried thyme

½ teaspoon dried marjoram

1 teaspoon vegan Worcestershire sauce

¼ teaspoon fine sea salt

¼ teaspoon ground black pepper

¼ teaspoon cayenne

4 cups fresh baby spinach

1 teaspoon gumbo filé

5 cups cooked brown rice

PER SERVING:

322 Calories

16 g Protein

12 g Total fat

4 g Saturated fat

0 g Monounsaturated fat

41 g Carbohydrates

7 g Fiber

3 g Sugar

169 mg Calcium

4 mg Iron

601 mg Sodium

Melt the margarine in a large stockpot or Dutch oven over medium to medium-low heat. Stir in the flour and cook, stirring constantly, until the flour paste becomes a deep caramel color, about 20 minutes.

Add the sausage, onion, celery, bell peppers, tomatoes, parsley, and garlic and cook, stirring often, until the vegetables begin to soften, about 4 to 5 minutes. Add the stock, bay leaves, thyme, marjoram, Worcestershire sauce, salt, black pepper, and cayenne. Bring to a boil and simmer over medium heat for 40 minutes, stirring occasionally. Stir in the spinach and filé and cook for an additional 5 minutes. Divide the rice among 10 serving bowls and ladle the gumbo over the rice.

One-Pot Jambalaya

MAKES 4 SERVINGS

While working on the Mardi Gras chapter of Quick and Easy Vegan Celebrations *I fell in love with the flavors of New Orleans. I never liked seafood, and I haven't eaten ham since I was a little girl, so most of the pork- and seafood-laden food of New Orleans just wasn't for me. But now that I've mastered the art of veganizing southern cuisine—most recently the dishes of New Orleans—I can't stop eating it! I have at least five gumbo recipes and four Jambalaya recipes in rotation at my house at all times. Here's one of my favorite one-pot jambalayas.*

2 tablespoons Earth Balance margarine

2 Andouille Sausage links, sliced thin (page 43)

½ medium onion, diced

3 celery stalks, diced

½ medium green bell pepper, diced

1 garlic clove, minced

4 bay leaves

¼ teaspoon fine sea salt

1 teaspoon ground white pepper

1 teaspoon dry mustard

½ teaspoon cayenne, optional

1 teaspoon gumbo filé

½ teaspoon ground cumin

1 teaspoon dried thyme

2 cups quick-cooking (10-minute) brown rice, uncooked

4 cups vegetable stock

PER SERVING:

331 Calories

17 g Protein

12 g Total fat

4 g Saturated fat

0 g Monounsaturated fat

42 g Carbohydrates

5 g Fiber

4 g Sugar

97 mg Calcium

3 mg Iron

1375 mg Sodium

Melt the margarine over medium-high heat in a Dutch oven or large heavy skillet, preferably cast iron. Add the sausage and cook for 3 minutes or until it begins to brown slightly. Add the onions, celery, bell pepper, and garlic and cook for 10 minutes or until vegetables are soft. Add the bay leaves, salt, white pepper, mustard, cayenne, gumbo filé, cumin, thyme, uncooked rice, and stock and stir. Bring to a boil then reduce the heat, cover, and simmer for 10 minutes. Uncover and cook for an additional 10 minutes or until most of the liquid has been absorbed. Remove the bay leaves before serving.

Baked Risotto

I have an obsession with risotto that borders on dangerous. Once I make a batch, I will eat it for breakfast, lunch, and dinner and even have it as a snack. The one thing that has kept my love affair with risotto at bay up to now is the time it takes, standing over a hot stove stirring and adding broth until the Arborio rice develops its rich, creamy risotto texture. My entire world changed when I happened across a recipe for baked risotto by Martha Stewart. Martha's version is a plain yet savory side dish or appetizer risotto that I have tweaked into a veganized, low-calorie main event, filled to the brim with fresh vegetables and flavor. Use leftovers to make Crispy Risotto Cakes (page 182).

MAKES 8 SERVINGS

1 tablespoon extra virgin olive oil

1¼ cups chopped leeks, rinsed

1½ cups Arborio rice

4 cups water

1 cup vegetable stock

1½ teaspoons dried basil

1½ teaspoons dried marjoram

¾ teaspoon fine sea salt

⅛ teaspoon freshly ground black pepper

1 large carrot, peeled and diced

1 large zucchini (about 12 ounces), diced

2 medium summer squash (about 12 ounces total), diced

2 tablespoons Earth Balance margarine

½ cup nutritional yeast

Preheat the oven to 425°F.

Warm the oil in an ovenproof saucepan or Dutch oven over medium heat. Add the leeks and cook until softened, about 2 minutes. Add the rice and cook, stirring to coat with oil, for 1 minute. Stir in 3 cups of the water and the stock, basil, marjoram, salt, black pepper, and carrot. Bring to a boil. Add the zucchini and summer squash and stir. Cover and transfer to the oven.

Bake until most of the liquid has been absorbed, 25 to 30 minutes. Remove from oven and stir in remaining 1 cup water and the margarine and nutritional yeast. Serve immediately.

PER SERVING:

184 Calories

8 g Protein

5 g Total fat

2 g Saturated fat

0 g Monounsaturated fat

38 g Carbohydrates

4 g Fiber

3 g Sugar

39 mg Calcium

1 mg Iron

344 mg Sodium

Crispy Risotto Cakes

MAKES 15 CAKES

I have a love affair with risotto that transcends the normal boundaries between food and love. Although I'm usually cooking for one I always make the full recipe for eight and either eat the whole thing as is over the course of just a couple days or split the batch in two, saving some to eat as traditional risotto and transforming the other half into these crisp yet creamy cakes that bake up quickly and pair well with Gingered Brussels Sprouts (page 111).

½ cup fresh bread crumbs (see Cook's Tip on page 184)

½ recipe Baked Risotto (page 181)

⅓ cup fresh basil, thinly sliced

Preheat the oven to 400°F. Line a baking sheet with foil and spray with cooking spray.

Put the bread crumbs into a shallow dish. Form the risotto into balls of approximately ¼ cup each, then flatten into patties and press into the bread crumbs to coat completely. Arrange on the prepared baking sheet and spray with cooking spray.

Bake for 30 minutes or until golden brown. Transfer the cakes to serving plates and top with the basil.

PER RISOTTO CAKE:

62 Calories

3 g Protein

2 g Total fat

0 g Saturated fat

0 g Monounsaturated fat

13 g Carbohydrates

1 g Fiber

1 g Sugar

30 mg Calcium

1 mg Iron

117 mg Sodium

Eggplant Parmesan

As I've said before, there are two ways I like eggplant: in Eggplant Fries (page 119) and in Eggplant Parmesan. A must-have for this recipe is fresh bread crumbs. Dried bread crumbs tend to fall off the eggplant when you coat it, but fresh bread crumbs absorb the moisture of the eggplant and create a beautiful golden crust around each eggplant slice as it bakes.

MAKES 6 SERVINGS

TOMATO SAUCE

1 tablespoon extra virgin olive oil

4 garlic cloves, minced

One 14-ounce can crushed tomatoes

1 tablespoon Italian seasoning

¼ teaspoon fine sea salt

EGGPLANT

Olive oil cooking spray

1¼ cups fresh bread crumbs (see Cook's Tip on page 184)

2 tablespoons plus 1½ teaspoons Parmesan Cheese (page 238)

1¼ teaspoons garlic powder

¼ teaspoon fine sea salt

¼ teaspoon ground black pepper

1 cup unsweetened plain almond milk or water

3 tablespoons Ener-G Egg Replacer

One 1-pound eggplant, cut into six ½-inch-thick slices

PER SERVING:

187 Calories

6 g Protein

6 g Total fat

1 g Saturated fat

1 g Monounsaturated fat

32 g Carbohydrates

6 g Fiber

3 g Sugar

186 mg Calcium

3 mg Iron

488 mg Sodium

To make the sauce:

Warm the oil in a medium saucepan over medium-high heat and sauté the garlic until fragrant, about 1 minute. Add the tomatoes, Italian seasoning, and salt. Bring to a low boil then lower the heat and cover. Simmer, stirring often, for 10 minutes.

To prepare the eggplant:

Preheat the oven to 400°F. Line a baking sheet with nonstick foil and spray lightly with olive oil cooking spray.

Combine the bread crumbs, Parmesan Cheese, garlic powder, salt, and black pepper in a shallow dish. Whisk together the milk and egg replacer in a small bowl. Dip each slice of eggplant into the milk mixture and then press into the bread crumb mixture to completely coat on both sides. Arrange the eggplant in a single layer on the prepared baking sheet and spray lightly with olive oil.

Bake for 20 minutes or until the bread crumbs are golden brown. To serve, divide the tomato sauce between 6 plates (about 2 to 3 tablespoons on each) and place an eggplant slice on top.

Cook's Tip: To create homemade fresh bread crumbs, pulse a hunk of day-old baguette or other crusty bread in a food processor until it breaks into small crumbs. Voilà!

White Bean Cassoulet

All you need on a cold winter's evening is a big bowl of White Bean Cassoulet, some crusty French bread, and a little olive oil to turn a good night into a great night.

MAKES 6 SERVINGS

2 tablespoons extra virgin olive oil

3 medium leeks, white parts only, rinsed and chopped

4 medium carrots, peeled and chopped

3 celery stalks, chopped

4 garlic cloves, minced

2 teaspoons dried thyme

½ teaspoon dried parsley

1 bay leaf

4½ cups cooked cannellini beans

4 cups vegetable stock

Fine sea salt

Freshly ground black pepper

Warm the oil in a large saucepan or Dutch oven over medium heat. Add the leeks, carrots, celery, and garlic and cook, stirring occasionally, until the vegetables have softened, about 15 minutes. Stir in the thyme, parsley, bay leaf, beans, and stock and bring to a low boil. Lower the heat, cover, and simmer until the carrots are tender, about 20 minutes.

Discard the bay leaf and mash some of the beans in the pan with the back of a spoon. Season with salt and black pepper.

PER SERVING:

258 Calories

11 g Protein

5 g Total fat

1 g Saturated fat

0 g Monounsaturated fat

43 g Carbohydrates

9 g Fiber

6 g Sugar

114 mg Calcium

4 mg Iron

1096 mg Sodium

Chickpea Cacciatore

It's scary how filling beans can be. They have the perfect combination of protein and fiber that releases glucose slowly into your blood stream and keeps you feeling full longer. Eating this cacciatore over brown rice or quinoa will leave you rubbing your belly in satisfaction but wishing you could have just one more bite.

One 28-ounce can whole plum or roma tomatoes, with juices

One 6-ounce can tomato paste

2 tablespoons extra virgin olive oil

3 garlic cloves, minced

½ cup diced white onion

1 medium carrot, peeled and diced

1 cup diced bell pepper of any color

2 teaspoons vegan Worcestershire sauce

2 teaspoons balsamic vinegar

Pinch of red pepper flakes

¼ teaspoon dried parsley

¼ teaspoon dried thyme

¼ teaspoon dried rosemary

1 teaspoon dried basil

1 teaspoon dried oregano

2½ cups cooked chickpeas

Freshly ground black pepper

PER SERVING:

219 Calories

9 g Protein

7 g Total fat

1 g Saturated fat

4 g Monounsaturated fat

34 g Carbohydrates

9 g Fiber

12 g Sugar

75 mg Calcium

4 mg Iron

288 mg Sodium

Put the tomatoes and tomato paste into a blender and blend until smooth.

Warm the oil in a large saucepan over medium-high heat. Add the garlic, onion, carrot, and bell pepper and sauté, stirring frequently to keep the garlic from burning, for 10 minutes or until carrots are tender. Add the tomato mixture to the pan along with the Worcestershire sauce, vinegar, red pepper flakes, parsley, thyme, rosemary, basil, and oregano. Allow the sauce to come to a low boil then reduce the heat, cover, and simmer for 20 minutes.

Add the chickpeas and cook for an additional 10 minutes. Season with black pepper.

Indian-Spiced Chickpeas

I'm still getting my feet wet when it comes to Indian food. One spice at a time, I'm beginning to understand the flavors of the country. This dish came together as I practiced with the spices and herbs of the region, throwing in a little of this and a little of that until the whole house smelled enchanting. If this doesn't sound like your idea of comfort food, just think of all those nights when you've come home late and ordered in takeout to eat curled up on the couch—sounds comforting to me!

MAKES 6 SERVINGS

2 tablespoons canola oil

½ cup diced white onion

2 garlic cloves, minced

1 tablespoon minced fresh ginger

½ teaspoon red pepper flakes

1½ cups vegetable stock

One 14.5-ounce can petite diced tomatoes, drained

3 cups cooked chickpeas

1½ teaspoons ground cumin

1½ teaspoons ground coriander

1½ teaspoons paprika

1 teaspoon ground turmeric

1 teaspoon garam masala

¼ teaspoon fine sea salt

3 cups cooked brown rice

Cook's Tip: **Garam means "hot" in Hindi, and this blend of ground spices popular in northern India will give a little extra warmth to any Indian-inspired dish. You can find this popular Indian spice in the spice aisle of your local grocery store or international market.**

Warm the oil in a medium saucepan over medium heat. Add the onion, garlic, and ginger and cook until the onions are translucent and the ginger is fragrant, about 3 to 4 minutes. Add the red pepper flakes and cook for an additional minute. Stir in the stock, tomatoes, chickpeas, cumin, coriander, paprika, and turmeric. Bring to a boil then reduce the heat to medium-low and stir in the garam masala and salt. Simmer for 5 to 10 minutes until the sauce has thickened. Serve over the brown rice.

PER SERVING:

311 Calories

10 g Protein

8 g Total fat

1 g Saturated fat

0 g Monounsaturated fat

51 g Carbohydrates

9 g Fiber

7 g Sugar

82 mg Calcium

4 mg Iron

332 mg Sodium

Kung Pao Tofu

MAKES 5 SERVINGS

I prefer roasted tofu's firmer texture in Asian foods, but roasting the tofu isn't essential. If you like the taste and texture of lightly pressed tofu, feel free to skip this step and just toss the pressed and cubed tofu into the sauce.

One 14-ounce package extra-firm tofu, drained, pressed (see Cook's Tip on page 39), and cut into ½-inch cubes

1 tablespoon canola oil

⅓ cup diced sweet onion

2 tablespoons minced fresh ginger

3 garlic cloves, minced

2 tablespoons mirin

2 tablespoons rice vinegar

2 tablespoons Bragg Liquid Aminos

2 tablespoons hoisin sauce

¼ cup agave nectar

¼ to ¾ teaspoon red pepper flakes

2½ cups cooked brown rice

1 pound broccoli, steamed

¼ cup chopped peanuts

PER SERVING:

327 Calories

14 g Protein

9 g Total fat

1 g Saturated fat

0 g Monounsaturated fat

48 g Carbohydrates

6 g Fiber

16 g Sugar

131 mg Calcium

2 mg Iron

539 mg Sodium

Preheat the oven to 425°F and line a baking sheet with parchment paper.

Spread the tofu cubes in a single layer on prepared baking sheet and bake until firm, about 15 to 20 minutes. While tofu is roasting, prepare the sauce.

Warm the oil in a medium saucepan over medium heat. Add the onion and cook until soft, about 3 minutes. Add the ginger and garlic and cook until fragrant, about 2 minutes, turning down the heat if necessary to avoid burning the garlic. Stir in the mirin and rice vinegar and simmer until they begin to reduce. Add the liquid aminos, hoisin sauce, agave nectar, and red pepper flakes and cook until the mixture begins to thicken slightly, about 2 minutes. Add the roasted tofu to the sauce and toss to coat.

Divide the rice among 5 serving plates and then divide the tofu, broccoli, and sauce evenly among the plates. Top with chopped peanuts.

Cook's Tip: Mirin is a sweet Japanese rice wine often used in cooking. You can find mirin down the ethnic or Asian aisle of your grocery store, where this is often stocked, sometimes under the name "rice wine."

Chik'n Curry

MAKES 4 SERVINGS

Usually I'm all about homemade seitan, but I've made an exception for my Chik'n Curry. Nothing matches the taste and texture of MorningStar Farms Meal Starters Chik'n Strips for this quick, easy, and light curry dish. They're high in protein, low in calories, and with the addition of curry and sweet golden raisins, big on flavor. If you've been scared to attempt curry, this is a great dish to start with.

3 tablespoons unbleached all-purpose flour

½ teaspoon fine sea salt

½ teaspoon cayenne

One 8-ounce package MorningStar Farms Meal Starters Chik'n Strips, defrosted

1 tablespoon canola oil

½ small onion, thinly sliced

2 garlic cloves, minced

1 tablespoon curry powder

1 cup water

⅓ cup golden raisins

1½ tablespoons ketchup

2 cups cooked quinoa

PER SERVING:

319 Calories

21 g Protein

8 g Total fat

1 g Saturated fat

0 g Monounsaturated fat

44 g Carbohydrates

5 g Fiber

11 g Sugar

68 mg Calcium

6 mg Iron

702 mg Sodium

Preheat the oven to 450°F and line a baking sheet with parchment paper.

Combine the flour, salt, and cayenne in a shallow dish or large sealable plastic bag. Add chik'n strips and toss to coat. Arrange the strips in a single layer on the prepared baking sheet. Spray with cooking spray and bake for 10 minutes or until slightly browned.

While the chik'n strips are baking, warm the oil in a medium saucepan over medium heat. Add the onion and garlic and cook for 2 to 3 minutes until the onions are translucent. Add the curry powder and stir until the onions are coated. Stir in the water, raisins, and ketchup and bring to a boil. Add the baked chik'n strips and simmer for 5 to 10 minutes until the sauce has thickened. Serve over the cooked quinoa.

Wangz

It's hard to resist frying up seitan nuggets and dipping them in hot sauce, but with a little help from panko bread crumbs, these Wangz are still spicy, crunchy, and deelish—even without the vat of hot oil.

MAKES 4 SERVINGS

1 cup unsweetened plain soy milk

½ cup hot sauce, plus more for dipping

1 tablespoon arrowroot powder

¾ cup panko bread crumbs

2 tablespoons unbleached all-purpose flour

¾ teaspoon paprika

1 teaspoon fine sea salt

¼ cup nutritional yeast

1½ teaspoons onion powder

½ teaspoon garlic powder

¼ teaspoon sugar

¼ teaspoon dried thyme

1 recipe Basic Seitan, shaped or cut into nuggets (page 41)

Preheat the oven to 400°F. Line a baking sheet with foil and spray with nonstick cooking spray.

Whisk together the milk, hot sauce, and arrowroot powder in a small bowl. In a shallow dish, combine the bread crumbs, flour, paprika, salt, nutritional yeast, onion powder, garlic powder, sugar, and thyme.

Dip each strip of seitan into the milk mixture and then press into the bread crumb mixture to coat on all sides, then dip into milk mixture again, and finally press back into the bread crumb mixture. Arrange on the prepared baking sheet. Spray with nonstick cooking spray and bake until crispy, about 25 to 30 minutes. Serve with extra hot sauce for dipping.

PER SERVING:

201 Calories

27 g Protein

3 g Total fat

0 g Saturated fat

0 g Monounsaturated fat

36 g Carbohydrates

7 g Fiber

4 g Sugar

112 mg Calcium

4 mg Iron

1375 mg Sodium

Gyros with Tzatziki Sauce

MAKES 4 GYROS

Tzatziki Sauce has become my new favorite all-purpose topping for just about everything. Even when I'm not making gyros I keep a little around for a dollop on Zucchini Fritters (page 116), Fried Green Tomatoes (page 118), or even Crispy Risotto Cakes (page 182).

TZATZIKI SAUCE

1 medium cucumber, peeled, seeded, and grated

½ small white onion, grated

1 cup plain soy yogurt

1½ teaspoons flax oil

2 teaspoons fresh lemon juice

¼ teaspoon fine sea salt

¼ teaspoon dried dill

½ teaspoon dried oregano

1 garlic clove, minced

Freshly ground black pepper to taste

GYROS

1 recipe Savory Seitan (page 42)

4 whole wheat pita pockets

1 large tomato, seeded and diced

To make the Tzatziki Sauce:

Combine all the ingredients in a medium bowl. Transfer to an airtight container and store in the refrigerator until ready to use, up to 4 days.

To make the gyros:

Preheat the oven to 400°F and line a baking sheet with nonstick foil or parchment paper.

Slice the seitan cutlets into thin slices and arrange on the prepared baking sheet. Bake until firm, about 10 minutes.

To assemble gyros, divide seitan and tomato between pita pockets evenly and top with Tzatziki Sauce.

PER GYRO:

288 Calories

25 g Protein

3 g Total fat

0 g Saturated fat

0 g Monounsaturated fat

49 g Carbohydrates

6 g Fiber

5 g Sugar

131 mg Calcium

4 mg Iron

967 mg Sodium

Seitan Cheesesteak

Cheesesteaks are evidence that it doesn't take a whole lot of fancy-schmancy ingredients to make a phenomenal sandwich. With just a little seitan, bell pepper, onion, and cheese sauce stuffed in a hoagie roll, you have one of the best sandwiches you will ever sink your teeth into, all for less than 300 calories. This sandwich appears in all its low-calorie, high-taste glory on the cover of this book, along with some oven-baked fries as featured in my Cheese Fries (page 120).

MAKES 4 CHEESESTEAKS

1 recipe Savory Seitan (page 42)

1 teaspoon canola oil

½ medium onion, thinly sliced

½ medium bell pepper of any color, thinly sliced

½ cup Classic Cheese Sauce (page 237) or Queso Dip (page 100)

4 hoagie rolls, about 85 calories each

Preheat the oven to 400°F and line a baking sheet with nonstick foil or parchment paper.

Cut the seitan cutlets into thin slices and arrange on the prepared baking sheet. Bake until firm, about 10 minutes.

While the seitan is baking, warm the oil in a medium skillet over medium heat. Add the onion and bell pepper and cook until the onions are translucent and the bell peppers soften, about 5 minutes.

Divide the baked seitan among the hoagie rolls and top with onion, bell pepper, and 2 tablespoons of cheese sauce each. Serve warm.

PER CHEESESTEAK,: USING CLASSIC CHEESE SAUCE

299 Calories

25 g Protein

6 g Total fat

1 g Saturated fat

0 g Monounsaturated fat

46 g Carbohydrates

6 g Fiber

4 g Sugar

114 mg Calcium

4 mg Iron

895 mg Sodium

Chik'n-Fried Seitan

If you are not familiar with the southern method of "chicken frying," it's not exactly what it sounds like. Unlike traditional southern-fried foods, there is no deep fryer involved. In fact, the whole art of "chicken frying" is in the flour coating and the thickness of the protein being fried. It requires thin pieces of protein, which is why you should cut each seitan cutlet in half. Then all you do is coat and pan-fry the cutlets, and you'll have a southern classic dish on your hands. Just don't forget the gravy!

SEITAN

1 recipe Basic Seitan, shaped into 4 cutlets (page 41)

¾ cup unbleached all-purpose flour

½ teaspoon fine sea salt

¼ teaspoon ground black pepper

½ teaspoon dried thyme

½ cup unsweetened plain almond milk

3 tablespoons Ener-G Egg Replacer

3 tablespoons canola oil

GRAVY

1½ cups vegetable stock

1 bay leaf

¼ cup nutritional yeast

1 tablespoon plus 1 teaspoon Bragg Liquid Aminos

½ teaspoon onion powder

1½ teaspoons dried sage

1 cup water

¼ cup unbleached all-purpose flour

PER SERVING:

145 Calories

13 g Protein

6 g Total fat

0 g Saturated fat

0 g Monounsaturated fat

20 g Carbohydrates

3 g Fiber

1 g Sugar

111 mg Calcium

2 mg Iron

663 mg Sodium

To fry the seitan:

Cut the seitan cutlets in half as you would a biscuit to create 8 thin cutlets.

Combine the flour, salt, black pepper, and thyme in a shallow dish. In a separate shallow dish whisk together the milk and egg replacer. Warm half the oil in a large skillet over medium-high heat.

One at a time, press 4 of the cutlets into the flour mixture to coat, dip into the milk mixture, press into the flour mixture again, and add to the hot skillet. Cook until each piece is browned on both sides, about 3 to 4 minutes per side. Repeat with remaining oil and cutlets. Arrange on serving plates.

To make the gravy:

Once the cutlets have been fried, add the stock, bay leaf, nutritional yeast, liquid aminos, onion powder, and sage to the skillet and whisk together until combined. Bring to a boil. Whisk together the water and flour in a small bowl and slowly whisk into the stock mixture. Reduce the heat to medium-low and simmer, stirring constantly, until the desired thickness is achieved. Remove the bay leaf.

Spoon warm gravy over each fried cutlet.

Chik'n Pot Pie

MAKES 12 SERVINGS

There's no getting around it—making pot pie is a long process, but thankfully it is super easy. Don't be intimidated by the long list of ingredients. Pot pies are made of simple, homey, classic ingredients that are staples in any good kitchen. So one Sunday afternoon, while you're sitting around the house watching old episodes of Law and Order, *try putting together this pot pie to pass the time. Although I typically don't use store-bought vegan meat analogues, Gardein makes an amazing cutlet called Chick'n Scallopini that goes perfectly in this pot pie and is easy on calories too. If you'd prefer, you can use a different mildly seasoned seitan, though the flavor (and nutritional data) won't be exactly the same.*

CRUST

- 2 cups unbleached all-purpose flour
- ¾ teaspoon fine sea salt
- 7 tablespoons Earth Balance margarine, softened and cut into pieces
- 3 to 4 tablespoons cold water

FILLING

- 1 tablespoon extra virgin olive oil
- ½ pound cremini mushrooms, chopped
- 1½ cups frozen pearl onions, thawed and patted dry
- 4 medium carrots, peeled and diced
- 3 cloves garlic, minced
- 3 tablespoons Earth Balance margarine
- ¼ cup plus 3 tablespoons unbleached all-purpose flour
- 2½ cups vegetable stock
- ¾ cup unsweetened plain soy milk
- 1 pound red potatoes, cut into ½-inch pieces
- 8 Gardein Chick'n Scallopini cutlets, thawed, patted dry, and chopped
- ¼ teaspoon fine sea salt
- ¼ teaspoon ground white pepper
- 1 cup frozen peas, thawed
- ¼ cup chopped fresh parsley
- 2 tablespoons fresh thyme
- 1 tablespoon Dijon mustard

PER SERVING:
341 Calories
16 g Protein
13 g Total fat
4 g Saturated fat
0 g Monounsaturated fat
39 g Carbohydrates
5 g Fiber
3 g Sugar
55 mg Calcium
5 mg Iron
861 mg Sodium

To make the crust:

Put the flour and salt in a food processor and pulse to combine. Add the margarine and pulse until the mixture resembles coarse cornmeal. Drizzle 3 tablespoons cold water over the mixture then pulse until the dough forms moist crumbs that are just beginning to clump together, adding more water if dough is too stiff.

Turn out the dough onto a large piece of plastic wrap. Shape the dough into a square then wrap tightly in the plastic and refrigerate until firm.

To make the filling:

While the dough is chilling, warm the oil in an 8-quart Dutch oven or stockpot over medium-high heat. Add the mushrooms and cook until well browned, 3 to 4 minutes. Add the onions and carrots and cook for an additional 5 to 6 minutes. Add the garlic and cook, stirring constantly, until fragrant, about 30 seconds more. Scrape the vegetables into a bowl and set aside.

Melt the margarine in the same pot over low heat. Add the flour and cook, whisking constantly, until the mixture becomes smooth, about 4 minutes. Slowly whisk in the stock and milk. Bring to a boil, whisking occasionally. Reduce the heat to low and add the potatoes, chopped cutlets, cooked vegetables, salt, and black pepper. Partially cover the pot and simmer until the potatoes and carrots are just tender, 15 to 18 minutes. Stir in the peas, parsley, thyme, and mustard.

Position a rack in the center of the oven and preheat to 425°F. Line a large baking sheet with foil.

Distribute the filling evenly among 12 ovenproof bowls or ramekins that hold about 1 cup each. Roll out the dough into a ⅛-inch-thick rectangle. With a round cookie cutter, cut 12 circles of dough that are slightly wider than the inner diameter of the bowls (if necessary, assemble the scraps and roll again). Cut a small X through the center of each circle. Top each bowl with a circle of dough. With your fingertips or the tip of a fork, gently press the dough against the edge of the bowl to seal.

Put the pot pies on the prepared baking sheet and bake until the filling is bubbling and the crust is deep golden-brown, about 45 minutes. Cool on a rack for 20 minutes before serving.

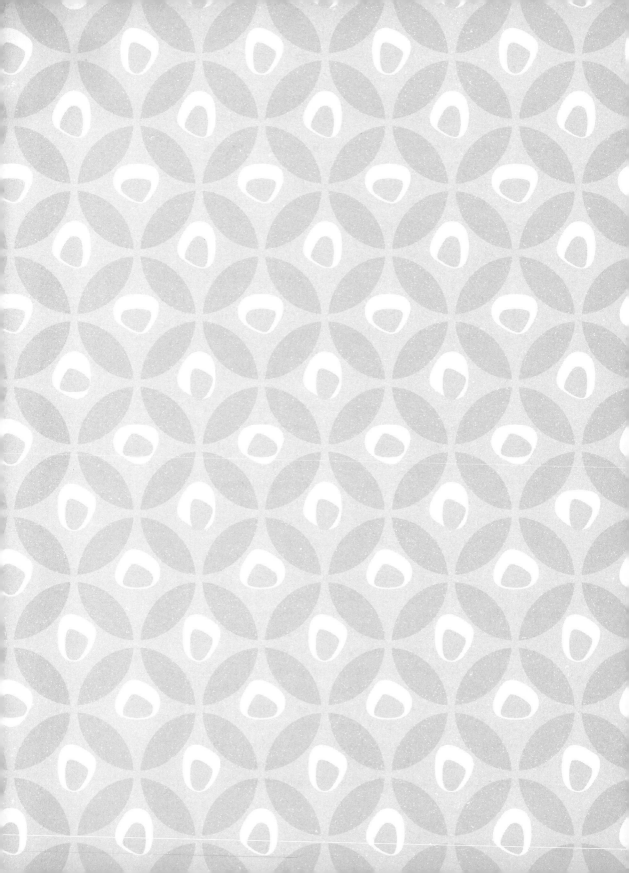

sinful sweets

NO MATTER WHAT you've been told, sugar is not the enemy. At only 15 calories a teaspoon it's hardly a high-calorie food. However, sugar is insanely delicious, and mixed with flour and margarine it's nearly irresistible. This irresistible combination is what leads many people to overindulge in desserts rather than putting them in their right place as occasional sweet treats to be enjoyed in moderation. To put it simply, one or two servings of Butter Pecan Ice Cream is great! Sitting down and eating one quart of Butter Pecan Ice Cream, not so great.

Butter Pecan Ice Cream

**MAKES 1 QUART
OR 8 SERVINGS**

Butter and cream—two words that have been banned from the vegan dictionary. I've done my best to bring them both back in a cruelty-free version—with this absolutely sinful vegan ice cream. I know it will be tough, but don't forget about portion control!

1½ cups plain soy yogurt

½ cup Grade A maple syrup

1 cup plain soy milk

1 teaspoon vanilla extract

¾ cup coarsely chopped pecans

Put the yogurt and maple syrup into a blender and blend until well combined. Add the milk and vanilla and pulse until combined.

Pour the mixture into an ice cream maker and process according to the manufacturer's directions, usually about 25 to 30 minutes. Add the pecans for the last 5 minutes of processing.

PER SERVING
(½ **CUP**):

173 Calories

4 g Protein

9 g Total fat

1 g Saturated fat

0 g Monounsaturated fat

21 g Carbohydrates

1 g Fiber

16 g Sugar

142 mg Calcium

1 mg Iron

20 mg Sodium

Cook's Tip: **Most of my ice cream recipes work best in an ice cream maker, so if you don't have one, satisfy your cool treat craving with some Pineapple-Mango Sorbet (page 204) or a Ruby Ice Pop (page 206) instead.**

Vanilla-Almond Ice Cream

I just love those little black specks of vanilla bean dotted throughout my ice cream. Whether it's store-bought or homemade, something about seeing those little flecks of black makes me feel like a little extra love went into making my ice cream—even if it is just as simple as scraping the seeds out of a vanilla bean.

1½ cups plain soy milk

½ cup sugar

1½ cups plain soy yogurt

½ teaspoon almond extract

1 vanilla bean, split lengthwise

Whisk together the milk and sugar until the sugar is completely dissolved. Add the yogurt and almond extract and whisk. Open the vanilla bean, scrape out the seeds with a spoon, and whisk the seeds into the mixture.

Pour the mixture into an ice cream maker and process according to the manufacturer's directions, usually about 25 to 30 minutes.

MAKES 1 QUART OR 8 SERVINGS

PER SERVING (½ CUP):

104 Calories

3 g Protein

2 g Total fat

0 g Saturated fat

0 g Monounsaturated fat

19 g Carbohydrates

1 g Fiber

17 g Sugar

141 mg Calcium

0 mg Iron

26 mg Sodium

Strawberry Cheesecake Ice Cream

MAKES 1 QUART OR 8 SERVINGS

If they're not in season, don't feel confined to using strawberries for this recipe. I haven't met a fresh-picked ripe fruit that doesn't taste fantastic in this ice cream.

One 8-ounce package vegan cream cheese

½ cup sugar

1 tablespoon fresh lemon juice

1 cup plain soy milk

½ pound fresh strawberries, chopped

Put the cream cheese, sugar, lemon juice, milk, and half the strawberries into a blender and blend until smooth. Pour into an airtight container and chill for at least 30 minutes. While the ice cream mixture is chilling, finely chop the remaining strawberries then cover and chill.

Pour the ice cream mixture into an ice cream maker and process according to the manufacturer's directions, usually about 25 to 30 minutes. Add the chopped strawberries for the last 5 minutes of processing.

PER SERVING
(½ CUP):
128 Calories
2 g Protein
5 g Total fat
2 g Saturated fat
0 g Monounsaturated fat
18 g Carbohydrates
1 g Fiber
15 g Sugar
42 mg Calcium
0 mg Iron
129 mg Sodium

Strawberry Jam Ice Cream

If you don't have time to make homemade Bread Machine Strawberry Jam to swirl into this ice cream, don't fret: any store-bought jar will work almost as well.

MAKES 1 QUART OR 8 SERVINGS

1½ cups plain soy milk

½ cup sugar

1½ cups plain soy yogurt

1 cup frozen strawberries, chopped

2 tablespoons Bread Machine Strawberry Jam (page 242) or strawberry preserves

Combine soy milk, sugar, soy yogurt, and strawberries in a blender and blend until smooth.

Pour the mixture into an ice cream maker and process according to the manufacturer's directions, usually about 25 to 30 minutes. In the last 5 minutes of processing slowly add in the strawberry jam.

PER SERVING

(½ **CUP**):

123 Calories

3 g Protein

2 g Total fat

0 g Saturated fat

0 g Monounsaturated fat

24 g Carbohydrates

1 g Fiber

20 g Sugar

145 mg Calcium

1 mg Iron

28 mg Sodium

Pineapple-Mango Sorbet

Typically I make ice creams and sorbets year-round, but Pineapple-Mango Sorbet is my one and only exception. There isn't a frozen or canned pineapple in the world that can compare to the taste of a freshly cut, in-season pineapple. Just the thought of one takes me back to summer instantly. I know it's hard, but try your best to wait until summer to try this sorbet. It'll reward you with the taste of sunshine in every sweet bite.

2½ cups frozen chopped mango

1½ cups water

½ cup agave nectar

¾ cup finely chopped fresh pineapple

Ice cream maker directions:

Put the mango, water, and agave nectar into a blender and blend until smooth. Scoop the mixture into an ice cream maker and process according to the manufacturer's directions, usually about 25 minutes. Add the chopped pineapple for the last 5 minutes of processing.

Freezer directions:

Put the mango, water, and agave nectar into a blender and blend until well combined.

Pour the mixture into a deep baking dish or a stainless steel bowl. Put the dish into your freezer until it begins to freeze around the edges, about 45 minutes, then stir thoroughly and return to freezer. Over the next two to three hours, continue checking and stirring every 30 minutes until the ice cream is frozen and creamy. Stir in the pineapple at the end.

PER SERVING
(½ CUP):
106 Calories
0 g Protein
0 g Total fat
0 g Saturated fat
0 g Monounsaturated fat
28 g Carbohydrates
1 g Fiber
27 g Sugar
9 mg Calcium
0 mg Iron
2 mg Sodium

Strawberry Sorbet Pops

Here in Georgia, blood oranges are only available for a couple weeks out of the year, so when I find them I try my best to incorporate them into anything and everything I can, including these Strawberry Sorbet Pops. If you can't find blood oranges, don't fret—regular orange juice will work just fine.

1½ pounds fresh strawberries

½ cup sugar

2 tablespoons fresh blood orange juice

Put the strawberries and sugar into a food processor and process until smooth. Add orange juice and pulse until combined. Pour the mixture into ½-cup popsicle molds. Freeze until firm, about 3 hours.

MAKES 8 ICE POPS

PER SERVING:

78 Calories

1 g Protein

0 g Total fat

0 g Saturated fat

0 g Monounsaturated fat

20 g Carbohydrates

2 g Fiber

17 g Sugar

14 mg Calcium

0 mg Iron

1 mg Sodium

Ruby Ice Pops

MAKES 8 ICE POPS

Why would anyone purchase store-bought ice pops when they can tranform three big juicy grapefruits, a little water, and some agave nectar into tangy-sweet ice pops in just a few hours?

2¾ cups fresh ruby grapefruit juice (about 3 grapefruits)

1 cup water

⅓ cup agave nectar

Combine all the ingredients and pour into eight ½-cup popsicle molds. Freeze until firm, about 3 hours.

PER ICE POP:
73 Calories
0 g Protein
0 g Total fat
0 g Saturated fat
0 g Monounsaturated fat
18 g Carbohydrates
0 g Fiber
11 g Sugar
8 mg Calcium
0 mg Iron
1 mg Sodium

Cherries Jubilee

When it comes to flambéing this classic dessert, the longer your match the better. For safety reasons, I recommend those long, 6- to 12-inch matches used for lighting fireplaces. Yes, it looks a bit dramatic holding a foot-long match above a saucepan of bubbling cherries, but safety first, my friends.

2 pounds fresh or frozen pitted bing cherries

¼ cup sugar

1 tablespoon cornstarch

¼ cup cherry brandy

¼ cup brandy

1 quart Vanilla-Almond Ice Cream (page 201)

Put the cherries, sugar, and cornstarch into a medium saucepan over medium heat. Cook, stirring constantly, until the sugar is completely dissolved. Bring to a boil and cook for 2 minutes.

Put the cherry brandy and regular brandy in a separate small saucepan over medium-high heat and heat until it begins to bubble slightly. Turn off the heat source or remove the pan from heat, light a match, and wave the match over the pan until the brandy lights. Lightly shake the pan to distribute the flame. The flame should subside on its own after about 30 seconds; if it doesn't, simply cover the saucepan with a lid.

Add the brandy mixture to the cherry mixture. Spoon into serving bowls with ice cream and serve immediately.

PER SERVING:

238 Calories

4 g Protein

2 g Total fat

0 g Saturated fat

0 g Monounsaturated fat

44 g Carbohydrates

3 g Fiber

38 g Sugar

155 mg Calcium

1 mg Iron

26 mg Sodium

Strawberry Shortcakes with Balsamic Syrup 📷

MAKES 8 SERVINGS

It's confession time again. I've had strawberry shortcakes for breakfast before. Not once, not twice—well, perhaps thrice, but let's keep that between us. I justify it to myself by calling it a breakfast food. Honestly, fluffy warm biscuits and fresh strawberries scream breakfast to me, but the moment you taste these you'll know I'm stretching the truth: they are pure dessert. But if you cheat and have one for breakfast, too, I won't tell a soul.

BISCUITS

2 cups unbleached all-purpose flour

¼ cup tablespoon sugar

2½ teaspoons baking powder

¼ teaspoon fine sea salt

½ cup Earth Balance margarine, chilled

1 cup plain almond milk, chilled

2 pounds fresh strawberries, hulled and quartered

¼ cup plus 3 tablespoons sugar

3 tablespoons balsamic vinegar

½ cup nondairy whipping cream, chilled

1 teaspoon vanilla extract

PER SERVING:

329 Calories

4 g Protein

13 g Total fat

6 g Saturated fat

0 g Monounsaturated fat

49 g Carbohydrates

3 g Fiber

22 g Sugar

96 mg Calcium

2 mg Iron

309 mg Sodium

Preheat the oven to 425°F and line a baking sheet with parchment paper.

Put the flour, ¼ cup of the sugar, the baking powder, and salt in a food processor and pulse to combine. Add the margarine and pulse until the mixture resembles coarse cornmeal. Add milk and pulse until moist clumps form. Transfer the dough to a lightly floured work surface. Gather the dough into ball then flatten into an 8 x 4-inch rectangle (about 1 inch thick). Cut the rectangle of dough lengthwise in half then crosswise into 4 equal strips to form 8 square biscuits. Transfer the biscuits to the prepared baking sheet and chill for 20 minutes.

Combine the strawberries, ¼ cup plus 1 tablespoon of the sugar, and the vinegar in medium bowl. Let stand for 30 minutes, stirring occasionally.

Remove the biscuits from refrigerator and sprinkle with 1 tablespoon of the sugar. Bake until golden brown and a toothpick inserted into the center of a biscuit comes out clean, about 15 minutes. Transfer to a rack to cool.

With an electric mixer, preferably with a whisking attachment, beat the whipping cream, vanilla, and the remaining 1 tablespoon sugar in a medium bowl until peaks form.

Cut the baked biscuits in half horizontally. Place the bottom half of each biscuit, cut side up, on a serving plate. Using a slotted spoon, divide the strawberries among biscuits. Spoon a dollop of whipped cream on top of the strawberries then cover each with the top half of the biscuit. Drizzle the leftover strawberry syrup over the biscuits or keep on the side for dipping.

Corn Flour Cupcakes
with Raspberry Buttercream Frosting

Cupcakes get a bad rap for being super high in calories and packed with excessive amounts of sugar. However, most homemade vegan cupcakes aren't that bad on the calorie and sugar scale. Topped off with frosting one of these cupcakes has the same amount of sugar as 6 ounces of vegan yogurt. Each of these cupcakes has only 14 grams of sugar, while there can be 18 to 22 grams of sugar in just 2 tablespoons of commercial frosting alone. But remember, these are a treat, not a meal. One cupcake won't have you tipping the scales but 5 or 6 will cause a bit of alarm, so exercise moderation (and generosity): eat one or two then share the rest with family and friends.

PER CUPCAKE
(WITHOUT FROSTING):

136 Calories

1 g Protein

6 g Total fat

1 g Saturated fat

0 g Monounsaturated fat

19 g Carbohydrates

1 g Fiber

8 g Sugar

59 mg Calcium

1 mg Iron

181 mg Sodium

PER CUPCAKE
(WITH FROSTING):

178 Calories

1 g Protein

8 g Total fat

2 g Saturated fat

0 g Monounsaturated fat

25 g Carbohydrates

1 g Fiber

14 g Sugar

59 mg Calcium

1 mg Iron

191 mg Sodium

CORN FLOUR CUPCAKES

⅔ cup unbleached all-purpose flour

⅔ cup corn flour

¾ cup confectioners' sugar

2 teaspoons baking powder

½ teaspoon fine sea salt

⅓ cup vegetable shortening

½ cup plain almond milk

¾ teaspoon vanilla extract

⅓ cup plain soy yogurt

RASPBERRY BUTTERCREAM FROSTING

1 tablespoon vegetable shortening

1 tablespoon Earth Balance margarine, softened

1 tablespoon raspberry jam or preserves

⅛ teaspoon almond extract

½ cup confectioners' sugar

To make the cupcakes:

Preheat the oven to 350°F and line a muffin pan with paper liners.

Stir together the all-purpose flour, corn flour, confectioners' sugar, baking powder, and salt until combined. Add the shortening, milk, vanilla, and yogurt and beat with an electric mixer at medium speed, scraping the mixture from the sides often, until just blended.

Divide the batter equally among the lined muffin cups. Bake for 20 to 22 minutes until a toothpick inserted into the center of a cupcake comes out clean. Let cool.

To make the frosting:

Beat together the shortening, margarine, jam, and almond extract with an electric mixer until thoroughly combined. Add the confectioners' sugar and whip until smooth.

Frost the cooled cupcakes using all the frosting.

Lemon Cornmeal Cake with
Lemon Glaze and Blueberry Sauce

This is my anytime pick-me-up cake. I'm not an emotional eater, but something about the process of making, baking, and eating this cake just lifts my spirits. Not only that, but this is one of my favorite cakes to share. I certainly can't eat 12 servings all by myself, so whenever I make this cake I usually slice it up, wrap up the pieces with a little blueberry sauce on the side, and give them to friends, co-workers, or classmates—just about anyone I come into contact with during the day. Seeing the look of joy on their faces lets me know that my spirit isn't the only one lifted by a good slice of cake made with love.

LEMON GLAZE

1½ cups confectioners' sugar

3 tablespoons fresh lemon juice

CAKE

1 cup plain almond milk

¼ cup vegan sour cream

¼ cup unsweetened applesauce

1 tablespoon lemon zest

¾ teaspoon vanilla extract

½ cup Earth Balance margarine, softened

¾ cup sugar

1 tablespoon plus 1 teaspoon baking powder

½ teaspoon fine sea salt

1½ cups unbleached all-purpose flour

⅓ cup cornmeal

BLUEBERRY SAUCE

3 cups fresh blueberries

⅔ cup light brown sugar

2 teaspoons fresh lemon juice

PER SERVING
(WITH GLAZE AND
BLUEBERRY SAUCE):

334 Calories

2 g Protein

9 g Total fat

3 g Saturated fat

0 g Monounsaturated fat

63 g Carbohydrates

2 g Fiber

43 g Sugar

144 mg Calcium

1 mg Iron

388 mg Sodium

To make the glaze:

Stir together confectioners' sugar and lemon juice in a small bowl until smooth. Set aside (don't refrigerate).

To make the cake:

Preheat the oven to 350°F and spray a 9-inch springform pan with nonstick cooking spray.

Whisk together the milk, sour cream, applesauce, lemon zest, vanilla, margarine, sugar, baking powder, and salt in a large bowl until combined. Add the flour and cornmeal and stir until smooth.

Pour the batter into the prepared springform pan. Bake 30 minutes or until a toothpick inserted into the center comes out clean. Run a knife around the edge of the hot cake and remove the sides of the pan. Gently remove the cake from the bottom piece of the pan if desired. While the cake is still hot, drop spoonfuls of the lemon glaze on top and gently spread with a knife or spatula. Allow cake to cool completely. While cake is cooling, make blueberry sauce.

To make the blueberry sauce:

Combine 1½ cups of the blueberries, the brown sugar, and lemon juice in a medium saucepan over medium heat. Stir until the sugar dissolves. Bring the mixture to a low boil and cook for about 5 minutes. Reduce heat to medium-low and simmer, stirring often, until the berries become soft and the sauce becomes syrupy, about 10 minutes. Remove from the heat and stir in the remaining 1½ cups blueberries. Using the back of a spoon, gently crush half the blueberries. Serve the sauce alongside the cake.

Moon Dusted Donuts

Being vegan keeps you from eating a lot of things that pack on the pounds when you're out on the town. For me, donuts are among them. I could eat a half-dozen donuts in a sitting if you let me. Thankfully, there aren't too many places around that offer vegan donuts, so when I have a craving for donuts I have to go home, pull up this recipe, and make them myself. Usually by the time the dough has risen I've eaten a nice meal and no longer have the impulse to eat six of them. Instead, I nibble on one donut and maybe a donut hole or two and am happy to leave the rest for another day.

2¼ teaspoons active dry yeast	⅛ teaspoon ground or freshly
2 tablespoons warm water	grated nutmeg
1½ teaspoons Ener-G Egg	⅛ teaspoon ground cinnamon
Replacer	3 tablespoons vegetable
2 tablespoons cold water	shortening
¾ cup plain almond milk	2¼ cups unbleached all-purpose
¼ cup sugar	flour, plus more for kneading
½ teaspoon fine sea salt	½ cup confectioners' sugar

Whisk the yeast into the warm water in a large bowl. Let stand for 5 minutes or until foamy. In a small bowl, whisk together the egg replacer and cold water.

Add the milk, sugar, salt, nutmeg, cinnamon, shortening, the egg replacer mixture, and 1 cup of the flour to the yeast mixture. Beat with an electric mixer on low speed for 1 minute. Beat in the remaining flour. Knead for 2 to 3 minutes until the dough is smooth and buoyant, adding more flour 2 tablespoons at a time as necessary to get this consistency. Return the dough to the bowl and cover with a damp paper towel. Set in a warm location and let stand until doubled in size, about an hour.

Turn out the dough onto a lightly floured surface and roll out to ½ inch thick. Cut out donuts with a donut cutter but make sure not to twist when pulling the cutter up. If you don't have a donut cutter, you can improvise by using a clean can to cut the outside circle and a knife to cut the inner, or even cut both circles with a knife, though your donuts won't be perfectly round. Set the donuts and donut holes aside, uncovered, and let double in size, about 20 minutes.

Preheat the oven to 420°F and line a baking sheet with parchment paper. Transfer the dough circles to the prepared baking sheet and bake for 8 to 10 minutes until golden. Sprinkle with confectioners' sugar.

Glazed Donuts

To whip up some glazed donuts, just follow the recipe for Moon Dusted Donuts and skip the step of dusting them with confectioners' sugar. Instead, dip each donut into one of these glazes. You can choose from Vanilla Glaze or Chocolate Glaze, or make a half-recipe of both glazes for a truly decadent batch.

1 recipe Moon Dusted Donuts (page 214)

VANILLA GLAZE

¼ cup plain almond milk

¼ teaspoon almond extract

½ teaspoon vanilla extract

2 cups confectioners' sugar

CHOCOLATE GLAZE

¼ cup plain almond milk

3 tablespoons unsweetened cocoa powder

¼ teaspoon almond extract

½ teaspoon vanilla extract

2 cups confectioners' sugar

Choose which glaze you would like to make. Whisk all the ingredients together in a medium bowl until smooth. Dip each donut and donut hole into the glaze and allow to cool.

MAKES 10 TO 12 DONUTS AND DONUT HOLES

PER DONUT AND DONUT HOLE WITH VANILLA GLAZE:

212 Calories

3 g Protein

3 g Total fat

1 g Saturated fat

43 g Carbohydrates

1 g Fiber

24 g Sugar

13 mg Calcium

1 mg Iron

100 mg Sodium

PER DONUT AND DONUT HOLE WITH CHOCOLATE GLAZE:

215 Calories

3 g Protein

4 g Total fat

1 g Saturated fat

2 g Monounsaturated fat

43 g Carbohydrates

1 g Fiber

24 g Sugar

15 mg Calcium

1 mg Iron

100 mg Sodium

Frosted Sugar Melt Cookies

MAKES 30 COOKIES

*Making the smallest change—adding feather-light confectioners'
sugar to cookies instead of granulated sugar—magically
transforms them into melt-in-your-mouth delights. Usually I like
to dip my cookies in a little almond milk, but be warned: these
cookies are so light and delicate they will disintegrate right in your
cup. So enjoy them as is—soft, frosted, and enchanting.*

COOKIES

1 cup confectioners' sugar

¾ cup Earth Balance margarine, softened

2 tablespoons plain almond milk

1 teaspoon vanilla extract

¼ teaspoon fine sea salt

2 teaspoons baking powder

½ teaspoon baking soda

½ teaspoon cream of tartar

1¾ cups unbleached all-purpose flour

FROSTING

1½ tablespoons Earth Balance margarine, softened

½ teaspoon vanilla extract

¾ cup confectioners' sugar

To make the cookies:

Preheat the oven to 350°F and line a baking sheet with parchment paper.

Cream the confectioners' sugar and margarine with an electric mixer. Add the milk, vanilla, salt, baking powder, baking
soda, and cream of tartar and beat to combine. Add the flour
½ cup at a time, beating between additions, until completely
incorporated.

Drop the dough by the tablespoon full onto the prepared
baking sheet. Bake for 10 to 12 minutes or until golden.

To make the frosting:

Beat together the margarine and vanilla with an electric mixer
until thoroughly combined. Add the confectioners' sugar and
whip until smooth.

Frost the cooled cookies using all the frosting.

**PER COOKIE
(WITH FROSTING):**

83 Calories

1 g Protein

4 g Total fat

2 g Saturated fat

0 g Monounsaturated fat

10 g Carbohydrates

0 g Fiber

4 g Sugar

21 mg Calcium

0 mg Iron

142 mg Sodium

Butter Rum Pound Cake

I can't think of too many things better than desserts that involve rum. This rich, buttery, fluffy pound cake pairs perfectly with its sugary sweet rum glaze. This one is definitely a crowd pleaser.

POUND CAKE

> 1 cup granulated sugar
>
> ½ cup Earth Balance margarine
>
> ¼ cup plain soy yogurt
>
> ¼ cup unsweetened applesauce
>
> ¾ teaspoon baking powder
>
> ¼ teaspoon baking soda
>
> ¼ teaspoon fine sea salt
>
> 1½ cups unbleached all-purpose flour
>
> ½ cup spiced rum

GLAZE (OPTIONAL)

> ½ cup confectioners' sugar
>
> 1 tablespoon spiced rum

To make the pound cake:

Preheat the oven to 350°F. Spray an 8 x 4-inch loaf pan with nonstick cooking spray.

Beat together the sugar, margarine, yogurt, and applesauce with an electric mixer for 2 to 3 minutes. Add the baking powder, baking soda, and salt and beat until incorporated. Add ½ cup flour then ¼ cup rum, beating between each addition, and repeat until all the flour and rum have been incorporated.

Scrape the batter into the prepared loaf pan and bake for 50 minutes or until a toothpick inserted into the center comes out clean. Cool the cake in the pan. While the cake is cooling, prepare glaze.

To make the glaze:

Stir together the confectioners' sugar and rum until smooth.

Run a knife around the edge of the cooled cake and remove from the loaf pan. Drizzle with glaze.

MAKES 12 SERVINGS

PER SERVING (WITHOUT GLAZE):

216 Calories

2 g Protein

8 g Total fat

3 g Saturated fat

2 g Monounsaturated fat

30 g Carbohydrates

1 g Fiber

17 g Sugar

29 mg Calcium

1 mg Iron

187 mg Sodium

PER SERVING (WITH GLAZE):

238 Calories

2 g Protein

8 g Total fat

3 g Saturated fat

2 g Monounsaturated fat

35 g Carbohydrates

1 g Fiber

22 g Sugar

29 mg Calcium

1 mg Iron

187 mg Sodium

Ooey Gooeys

MAKES 20 ROLLS

The name says it all—these are ooey, gooey cinnamon rolls dripping with frosting and laced with goodness. Using a bread machine will cut down on your prep time considerably, but even without one these are far from labor intensive: you will spend the bulk of the preparation time waiting for the dough to rise. Ooey Gooeys aren't necessarily quick to make, but despite the long list of ingredients they are incredibly easy—and, I think you'll agree, worth the wait.

DOUGH

1 tablespoon active dry yeast

1¼ cup plain almond milk, warm if making dough by hand

½ cup granulated sugar

½ cup Earth Balance margarine, softened

½ teaspoon fine sea salt

¼ cup instant mashed potato flakes

3 cups unbleached all-purpose flour

1 cup whole wheat pastry flour

FILLING

½ cup packed light brown sugar

⅛ teaspoon ground allspice

2 tablespoons ground cinnamon

1½ teaspoons canola oil

OOEY GOOEY DRIZZLE

¼ cup Earth Balance margarine, softened

¾ cup confectioners' sugar

2 tablespoons vegan cream cheese

1 tablespoon plain almond milk

¼ teaspoon vanilla extract

To make the dough in a bread machine:

Put all of the ingredients for the rolls into a bread machine according to the manufacturer's directions and choose the dough cycle (use the 2-pound setting).

PER ROLL:

220 Calories

3 g Protein

8 g Total fat

3 g Saturated fat

0 g Monounsaturated fat

35 g Carbohydrates

2 g Fiber

15 g Sugar

21 mg Calcium

2 mg Iron

141 mg Sodium

QUICK AND EASY LOW-CAL VEGAN COMFORT FOOD

To make the dough by hand:

Sprinkle the yeast over the warm milk in a large bowl and allow to dissolve. Add the sugar, margarine, salt, potato flakes, all-purpose flour, and pastry flour and stir to mix well. Dust your hands lightly with flour and form the dough into a large ball. Return the dough to the bowl and cover with a damp towel. Set in a warm place and let stand until doubled in size, about 1 hour.

Once the dough has risen, turn out onto a lightly floured surface and roll out to ¼ inch thickness.

Preheat the oven to 400°F. Line a baking sheet with parchment paper.

To make the filling:

Combine the brown sugar, allspice, and cinnamon in a small bowl.

Spread the oil over the surface of the rolled-out dough, then sprinkle evenly with the brown sugar. Starting from one of the longer sides, carefully roll up the dough. Cut the dough into 1½-inch slices and arrange, cut side down, on the prepared baking sheet.

Bake for 10 minutes or until light golden brown. While the rolls are baking, prepare the Ooey Gooey Drizzle.

To make the drizzle:

Put all the ingredients into a medium bowl and beat with an electric mixer on high until fluffy.

When the rolls are done, drizzle icing over each roll.

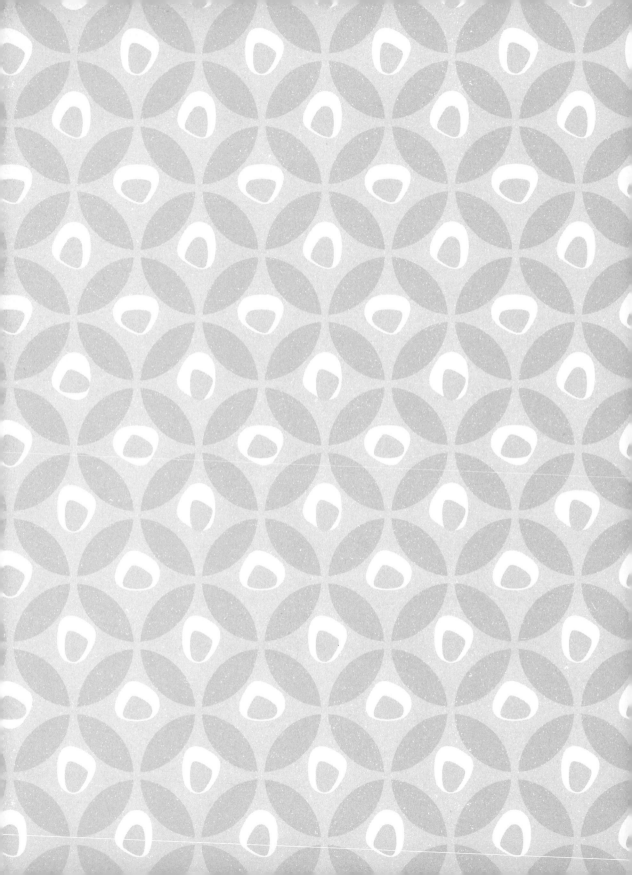

Beverages

LIQUID CALORIES IN the form of sodas, your morning overpriced latte, and even fruit juices are the quickest ways to inject hidden unnecessary calories into the diet. Typically beverages don't fill you up like food does, and they also typically lack any real nutritional benefit. But just like desserts, they have their place in a healthy diet—it's all about being mindful of what you're drinking and how it contributes to your overall caloric load for the day. These beverages help pack a nutrition-rich punch while also satisfying your sweet tooth. Not only that, but they are fun to make and share with friends and family.

Sugar-Full Pomegranate Lemonade

MAKES 6 CUPS

I am not a fan of sugar substitutes. Sugar only has 15 calories per teaspoon, and I'd rather have the sweet taste of pure cane sugar on my tongue any day than the bitter or sour aftertaste of fake sugar.

¾ cup pomegranate juice

1 cup fresh lemon juice (about 4 large lemons)

4 cups cold water

¾ cup sugar

Stir all the ingredients together in a 2-quart pitcher until the sugar dissolves. Serve over ice.

PER SERVING
(1 CUP):
124 Calories
0 g Protein
0 g Total fat
0 g Saturated fat
0 g Monounsaturated fat
33 g Carbohydrates
0 g Fiber
26 g Sugar
10 mg Calcium
0 mg Iron
6 mg Sodium

Watermelon-Basil Mock Mojito

Writing this book and writing Quick and Easy Vegan Celebrations *were two very different experiences for me. For* Quick and Easy Vegan Celebrations *I got to rummage through my liquor and liqueur cabinets and create cocktails for every occasion. However, because I've been pregnant through the entire process of writing this book, the drinks this time around are all fizzy, sweet, and alcohol free. This one, Watermelon-Basil Mock Mojito, was my signature drink of the summer. The sweetness is out of this world, although it needs almost no sugar at all. By the way, if you're ever lucky enough to find yellow watermelon, I implore you, you must try it in this mojito!*

MAKES TWO 16-OUNCE
SERVINGS

4 cups cubed fresh watermelon (about 1 pound)

6 fresh basil leaves

1½ teaspoons grated fresh ginger

1 tablespoon plus 1 teaspoon sugar

1 tablespoon plus 1 teaspoon fresh lime juice

Sparkling water or club soda

Put the watermelon into a blender and blend until smooth. Set aside.

Divide the basil, ginger, sugar, and lime juice between two 16-ounce glasses. Muddle the ingredients with a spoon until the sugar has dissolved. Divide the blended watermelon between the glasses then top off with sparkling water until the glasses are filled.

Cook's Tip: For a stronger ginger taste, add the ginger to the blender along with the watermelon and blend until smooth.

PER SERVING:

134 Calories

2 g Protein

1 g Total fat

0 g Saturated fat

0 g Monounsaturated fat

34 g Carbohydrates

2 g Fiber

28 g Sugar

67 mg Calcium

2 mg Iron

4 mg Sodium

Home-Brewed Ginger Ale

MAKES FIVE 16-OUNCE SERVINGS

Soda. It's something so simple to make, yet because most of our soda comes to us premixed and made with a list of mystery ingredients and hidden flavors, it's become quite mysterious. Use this mystique to your advantage when making Home-Brewed Ginger Ale for a party. In reality, the process of making homemade ginger ale is as easy as throwing three ingredients into a pot, letting it simmer for an hour, then straining it and stirring in a little club soda. But don't tell your friends that. Let them think that you hold the keys to the mystical world of soda making when you serve this treat at your next party.

7 to 8 ounces unpeeled fresh ginger, washed and chopped

1½ cups sugar

4 cups water

4 cups club soda

Put the ginger into a food processor and pulse until minced. Transfer to a medium saucepan and add the sugar and water. Bring to a boil then reduce the heat and simmer, uncovered, for 1 hour, stirring occasionally. Let cool.

Strain the syrup through a large fine-mesh sieve over a large bowl, pressing the ginger against the sides of the sieve to squeeze out the last bits of flavor. Discard the ginger.

To make a glass of ginger ale, gently stir together 1 cup of the club soda and ⅓ cup of the ginger syrup in a 16-ounce glass then add ice to fill.

PER SERVING:
270 Calories
1 g Protein
0 g Total fat
0 g Saturated fat
0 g Monounsaturated fat
69 g Carbohydrates
1 g Fiber
61 g Sugar
12 mg Calcium
0 mg Iron
10 mg Sodium

Lemongrass Soda

Right now there is an entire shelf in my freezer dedicated to Lemongrass Soda syrup. I rarely drink soda, but I can't stop making the base syrup for this recipe. The combination of lemongrass and ginger is so robustly aromatic that it fills your whole house with a scent you can almost taste. It's better than any scented candle ever invented, and in the end you get five big servings of Lemongrass Soda. Not a bad deal.

MAKES FIVE 16-OUNCE SERVINGS

½ cup thinly sliced peeled ginger

3 fresh lemongrass stalks, split lengthwise and cut into 1-inch pieces

2 cups water

1 cup sugar

3 tablespoons fresh lemon juice

5 cups club soda or sparkling water

Combine the sliced ginger with the lemongrass and water in a medium saucepan and bring to a boil. Stir in the sugar. Reduce the heat, cover, and simmer for 30 minutes.

Strain the syrup through a fine-mesh sieve over a large bowl. Discard the ginger and lemongrass pieces. Stir in the lemon juice.

For each glass of soda, gently stir together ¼ cup of the lemongrass syrup and 1 cup of the club soda in a 16-ounce glass then add ice to fill.

PER SERVING:

179 Calories

0 g Protein

0 g Total fat

0 g Saturated fat

0 g Monounsaturated fat

46 g Carbohydrates

0 g Fiber

41 g Sugar

25 mg Calcium

1 mg Iron

54 mg Sodium

Pumpkin Seed Milk

MAKES 4 CUPS

This milk is surprisingly subtle in flavor and goes well in everything from a venti latte to chocolate chip cookies. Pumpkin seeds are also an excellent source of protein, iron, and zinc.

1 cup raw pumpkin seeds

4 cups water

2 tablespoons agave nectar

¼ to ½ teaspoon vanilla extract or pulp from ½ vanilla bean (optional)

Put the pumpkin seeds and ¾ cup of the water into a blender and blend until smooth. Add the agave nectar and vanilla, then, with the blender running, *slowly* add the remaining water. Store for up to 4 days in an airtight container in the refrigerator.

PER SERVING
(1 CUP):
217 Calories
8 g Protein
16 g Total fat
3 g Saturated fat
0 g Monounsaturated fat
14 g Carbohydrates
1 g Fiber
8 g Sugar
20 mg Calcium
5 mg Iron
11 mg Sodium

Pepita Smoothie

Using raw pepitas instead of soy or almond milk as the base of this smoothie gives the smoothie that little extra bit of fat that makes it super filling and that will keep you satisfied long after one of those mall-brand smoothies would have left you hanging.

MAKES TWO 8-OUNCE SMOOTHIES

¼ cup raw pumpkin seeds

1 cup water

1 tablespoon agave nectar

1 cup frozen mango

1 cup frozen strawberries

Combine all ingredients in a high-speed blender and blend until smooth.

PER SMOOTHIE:

201 Calories

5 g Protein

8 g Total.fat

2 g Saturated fat

0 g Monounsaturated fat

31 g Carbohydrates

4 g Fiber

24 g Sugar

30 mg Calcium

3 mg Iron

8 mg Sodium

Strawberry Milk Shake 📷

**MAKES FOUR 8-OUNCE
MILK SHAKES**

A milk shake? In a low-calorie cookbook?! Oh yes! When I said that I don't believe in using fake ingredients to keep the calories down, I meant it. This strawberry milk shake is all about putting fresh strawberries on display, from the base of Strawberry Jam Ice Cream to the frozen strawberries that make it nice and thick to the soy milk that gives it that velvety smooth texture.

4 cups Strawberry Jam Ice Cream (page 203)
½ cup frozen strawberries
2 cups plain soy milk

Put all the ingredients into a blender and blend until smooth.

PER MILK SHAKE:

302 Calories
10 g Protein
6 g Total fat
0 g Saturated fat
0 g Monounsaturated fat
53 g Carbohydrates
3 g Fiber
44 g Sugar
442 mg Calcium
2 mg Iron
115 mg Sodium

Mexican Hot Cocoa 📷

I'm not a huge fan of chocolate, but I can't resist the taste and smell of Mexican chocolate. The notes of almond, cinnamon, and vanilla with just a hint of spice from cayenne pepper take my taste buds to another world. Be careful with the cayenne, though: with such a sweet base underneath it, the heat jumps out quick. If you aren't paying attention when you add that dash, you will have one spicy hot cocoa on your hands!

¼ cup unsweetened cocoa powder

¼ cup plus 1 tablespoon agave nectar

¾ teaspoon ground cinnamon

4 cups unsweetened plain almond milk

¾ teaspoon vanilla extract

½ teaspoon almond extract

Dash of cayenne

Whisk all the ingredients together in a medium saucepan and heat over medium heat until warmed through.

MAKES FOUR 8-OUNCE SERVINGS

PER SERVING:

132 Calories

2 g Protein

4 g Total fat

0 g Saturated fat

0 g Monounsaturated fat

25 g Carbohydrates

3 g Fiber

20 g Sugar

462 mg Calcium

2 mg Iron

181 mg Sodium

Sauces, Spreads, and Spice Blends

IT'S THE LITTLE touches that really make the difference in home cooking. Serving up homemade jams and jellies with fresh baked biscuits or whipping up a batch of enchilada sauce from scratch to make Wet Burritos (page 176) shows that a little extra love, time, and care went into making a dish. Plus, making your own sauces, spreads, and spice blends allows you to stay in complete control of what is in the food you eat. It's surprising how many ingredients are on the back of a jar of jelly these days when all it takes is a little sugar, fruit, and pectin. The very best part about making your own sauces, spreads, and spice blends is that they are incredibly quick and easy to make.

Spiced Ketchup 📷

This ketchup is dressed to impress with an inventive mix of herbs and seasonings that turn regular ole ketchup into a gourmet experience. Keeps for about a week in the refrigerator.

¾ cup ketchup

½ teaspoon ground coriander

¼ teaspoon dry mustard

⅛ teaspoon ground ginger

¼ teaspoon cayenne

¼ teaspoon ground cloves

¼ teaspoon ground allspice

Whisk all the ingredients together. Cover and keep refrigerated until ready to use.

PER SERVING
(1 TABLESPOON):

15 Calories

0 g Protein

0 g Total fat

0 g Saturated fat

0 g Monounsaturated fat

4 g Carbohydrates

0 g Fiber

3 g Sugar

3 mg Calcium

0 mg Iron

167 mg Sodium

Sweet Caroline BBQ Sauce

MAKES 2½ CUPS

When I lived in South Carolina, the fact that I didn't eat meat was a source of great dismay to just about anyone I ran into. "So, you don't eat barbecue?!" would always be their first question—or perhaps accusation. In South Carolina barbecue means one thing and one thing only—pork, pork, and more pork slathered in sweet vinegary barbecue sauce. I only lived in South Carolina for 2½ years and 6 days (but who's counting?), and in that amount of time I learned more about barbecue and barbecue culture than any one person really needs to know in a lifetime. I learned the nuances of ketchup-based, mustard-based, and vinegar-based sauces as well as the ultra-spicy vinegar and pepper mix, and over the years I have perfected my version of a ketchup-based Carolina barbecue sauce. There's just a touch of vinegar and a sweetness provided almost entirely by apple cider. This is sweet vinegary goodness to do any Carolinian proud.

1 teaspoon canola oil

⅔ cup diced sweet onion

2 garlic cloves, smashed and minced

1½ cups ketchup

1½ cups apple cider

¼ cup Grade A maple syrup

1 tablespoon apple cider vinegar

1 tablespoon vegan Worcestershire sauce

¼ teaspoon ground black pepper

⅛ teaspoon cayenne

Warm the oil in a medium saucepan over medium heat. Add the onion and sauté until soft, about 2 minutes. Add the garlic and cook until fragrant, about 1 minute. Stir in the ketchup, apple cider, maple syrup, vinegar, Worcestershire sauce, black pepper, and cayenne. Bring to a low boil then reduce the heat and simmer, uncovered, until the sauce begins to thicken and is slightly reduced, about 15 to 20 minutes.

PER SERVING
(¼ CUP):
84 Calories
1 g Protein
1 g Total fat
0 g Saturated fat
0 g Monounsaturated fat
20 g Carbohydrates
1 g Fiber
17 g Sugar
18 mg Calcium
0 mg Iron
442 mg Sodium

Taco Seasoning Mix

Store-bought taco seasoning mixes tend to have lots of mystery ingredients, some of which are initials instead of whole words. I prefer not to have to dust off my 1989 set of Encyclopaedia Britannicas *just to figure out what compounds are hidden in my seasonings. I just whip up a double or triple batch of this mix and keep it in the pantry so it's there whenever I need it.*

3 tablespoons chili powder

1 teaspoon garlic powder

1 teaspoon onion powder

¼ teaspoon cayenne or red pepper flakes

2 teaspoons paprika

2 tablespoons ground cumin

1 teaspoon dried oregano

1 teaspoon fine sea salt

½ teaspoon ground black pepper

Mix together all the ingredients in a small bowl. Store in an airtight container.

PER SERVING
(1 TABLESPOON):
22 Calories
1 g Protein
1 g Total fat
0 g Saturated fat
0 g Monounsaturated fat
4 g Carbohydrates
2 g Fiber
1 g Sugar
30 mg Calcium
2 mg Iron
373 mg Sodium

Ancho Chile Sauce

Ancho Chile Sauce provides the robust flavor base for southwest recipes like Plantain and Black Bean Tamales (page 174), Pinto Beans in Ancho Chile Sauce (page 168), and Refried Black Beans (page 113). It's big on flavor, small on calories and, incidentally, incredibly high in vitamin A—700 IU per tablespoon.

2 dried ancho chiles

1½ cups boiling water

½ medium white or yellow onion, chopped

1 garlic clove

2 teaspoons ground cumin

½ teaspoon fine sea salt

Pour the boiling water over the chiles in a small bowl and soak until the chiles have softened, about 30 minutes. Remove the chiles from the water and put into a food processor along with the onion, garlic, cumin, salt, and ½ cup of the soaking water. Process until smooth. Store in an airtight container in the refrigerator for up to 1 week.

MAKES ⅔ CUP

PER SERVING
(1 TABLESPOON):

14 Calories

1 g Protein

0 g Total fat

0 g Saturated fat

0 g Monounsaturated fat

3 g Carbohydrates

1 g Fiber

0 g Sugar

8 mg Calcium

1 mg Iron

120 mg Sodium

Enchilada Sauce

MAKES 3 CUPS

If you're not going to be using this sauce right away, you can store it in the freezer for up to 3 months so it'll be there for you when you're ready to make enchiladas or Wet Burritos (page 176).

3 cups vegetable stock

1½ tablespoons chili powder

½ teaspoon ground cumin

½ teaspoon garlic powder

½ teaspoon dried oregano

¼ teaspoon ground black pepper

1 cup tomato sauce

¼ cup unbleached all-purpose flour

Put 2½ cups stock, chili powder, cumin, garlic powder, oregano, black pepper, and tomato sauce in a medium saucepan and bring to a low boil. Reduce heat, cover, and simmer for 10 minutes, stirring occasionally.

Whisk together the flour and the remaining ½ cup of stock in a small bowl and add to the enchilada sauce. Simmer for 5 minutes or until the desired consistency is reached.

Use immediately or transfer to an airtight container and store in the refrigerator for up to 5 days.

PER SERVING
(1 CUP):

94 Calories

3 g Protein

1 g Total fat

0 g Saturated fat

0 g Monounsaturated fat

20 g Carbohydrates

3 g Fiber

6 g Sugar

29 mg Calcium

2 mg Iron

1,017 mg Sodium

Classic Cheese Sauce

This cheese sauce goes on everything from Seitan Cheesesteak (page 193), Cheese Fries (page 120), Chili Cheese Fries (page 165), and Chili Cheese Dogs (page 164) to baked potatoes or broccoli.

MAKES 2½ CUPS

1 medium Yukon Gold potato, scrubbed and diced

1 medium carrot, peeled and diced

½ cup diced white onion

1 garlic clove, chopped

1 cup water

¾ teaspoon fine sea salt

2 teaspoons lemon juice

½ cup cashews

Combine the potato, carrot, onion, garlic, and water in a small saucepan over medium heat. Bring to a boil then lower the heat, cover, and simmer for 10 minutes or until the vegetables are tender. (The smaller you cut the vegetables, the less time they will take to cook.)

Put the salt, lemon juice, cashews, and the cooked vegetables into a blender along with the cooking water and blend until completely smooth.

PER SERVING
(½ CUP):
107 Calories
3 g Protein
5 g Total fat
0 g Saturated fat
0 g Monounsaturated fat
13 g Carbohydrates
1 g Fiber
3 g Sugar
16 mg Calcium
1 mg Iron
366 mg Sodium

Parmesan Cheese

One of my favorite brands of vegan Parmesan cheese is Parma! I love it because the ingredients are simple: walnuts, nutritional yeast, and love. I'd been buying Parma! for years before one day it occurred to me: I have walnuts, nutritional yeast, and love right here in my own kitchen. I decided to play around with the various nuts that I keep on hand, and I remixed the Parma! formula to include cashews, almonds, and nutritional yeast along with just a hint of salt and a whole lot of love.

¾ cup raw cashews

¼ cup raw almonds

3 tablespoons nutritional yeast

½ teaspoon fine sea salt

Add all ingredients to a food processor and process until mixture resembles a light cornmeal. Store, refrigerated, in an airtight container for up to a week.

PER SERVING
(1 TABLESPOON):

43 Calories

2 g Protein

4 g Total fat

0 g Saturated fat

0 g Monounsaturated fat

3 g Carbohydrates

1 g Fiber

0 g Sugar

8 mg Calcium

1 mg Iron

75 mg Sodium

Cook's Tip: You can soak the nuts for a few hours if you'd like them to yield a creamier texture, or you can just use plain raw nuts—either way, the result will be delicious.

Frenchy Dressing

MAKES 1½ CUPS OR
12 SERVINGS

I can't imagine the French putting ketchup in anything, let alone a salad dressing, but I'm a country girl at heart, and I love to sneak ketchup into any dish I can think of. I'm not saying that I'm obsessed with ketchup or anything, but let's just say that I may or may not buy it in bulk. French dressing is a quick and easy way to gussy up a plain salad, and this Frenchy Dressing is a spin on the old classic.

¼ cup plus 2 tablespoons apple cider vinegar

½ cup plus 2 tablespoons ketchup

1 tablespoon agave nectar

1 teaspoon vegan Worcestershire sauce

½ teaspoon paprika

Pinch of cayenne

Pinch of ground white pepper

½ teaspoon onion powder

½ cup canola oil

1 garlic clove, pressed and minced

Put vinegar, ketchup, agave nectar, Worcestershire sauce, paprika, cayenne, white pepper, and onion powder into a blender and blend on medium speed until combined. Turn the blender speed down to low and slowly add the oil to incorporate. Transfer to an airtight container and stir in the garlic. Cover and keep refrigerated for up to a week.

PER SERVING
(1 OUNCE):

100 Calories

0 g Protein

9 g Total fat

1 g Saturated fat

0 g Monounsaturated fat

5 g Carbohydrates

0 g Fiber

4 g Sugar

4 mg Calcium

0 mg Iron

150 mg Sodium

South Carolina Peach Jam

I've lived in Georgia for six years and have yet to see one peach tree, but when I lived in South Carolina peach trees were everywhere. That's where I experienced the sweetest, juiciest peaches I have ever had in my life. Coincidentally, when the summer rolls around in Georgia, farmers' markets are filled with South Carolina peaches. I try to take advantage of the cheap seasonal prices and use these sweet peaches in everything I can think of, from cobblers to jams. Here's my favorite way to convert 3 pounds of peaches into a spiced summer jam. One of the advantages of using seasonal fruits is that you don't need to add nearly as much sugar, and because this jam freezes well, you can use it all year-round.

3 pounds fresh ripe peaches, peeled and finely diced

2 tablespoons fresh lemon juice

2 cups sugar

3 tablespoons fruit pectin

2 teaspoons grated fresh ginger

½ teaspoon ground mace

¼ teaspoon ground cinnamon

Sterilize 3 pint jars.

To make on the stove:

Combine the peaches, lemon juice, and sugar in a medium saucepan over medium heat and bring to a low boil. Stir in the pectin and return to a boil. Add the ginger, mace, and cinnamon and continue to boil, stirring constantly, for 1 minute.

Remove the hot jam from the heat and pour into the sterilized jars, leaving a ¼-inch space between the top of the jam and the neck of the jar. Cover and seal according to the jar manufacturer's directions. Let sit, undisturbed, for 24 hours to set.

PER SERVING
(1 TABLESPOON):

22 Calories

0 g Protein

0 g Total fat

0 g Saturated fat

0 g Monounsaturated fat

6 g Carbohydrates

0 g Fiber

5 g Sugar

1 mg Calcium

0 mg Iron

0 mg Sodium

To make in a bread machine:

Combine all the ingredients in a large bowl and transfer to a bread machine. Process according to the manufacturer's directions.

Pour the hot jam into the sterilized jars, leaving a ¼-inch space between the top of the jam and the neck of the jar. Cover and seal according to the jar manufacturer's directions. Let sit, undisturbed, for 24 hours to set.

Bread Machine Strawberry Jam

MAKES 1½ CUPS

Homemade jam is so simple to make I can't believe there was ever a time when I used the store-bought stuff. Homemade jams and jellies also make wonderful gifts. You could never wrap up a jar of commercial grape jelly and give it to your in-laws, but wrap up a jar of Bread Machine Strawberry Jam and they'll think you're the most wonderful son- or daughter-in-law in the world.

1 pound hulled fresh strawberries
⅔ cup sugar
1 tablespoon fresh lemon juice
1 teaspoon fruit pectin

Put the strawberries, sugar, and lemon juice into a food processor and pulse until the strawberries are broken down a bit (there should be some medium-size pieces). Add the pectin and pulse to combine. Transfer the mixture to a bread machine, choose the jelly/jam setting, and process according to the manufacturer's directions.

PER SERVING
(1 TABLESPOON):
28 Calories
0 g Protein
0 g Total fat
0 g Saturated fat
0 g Monounsaturated fat
7 g Carbohydrates
0 g Fiber
6 g Sugar
3 mg Calcium
0 mg Iron
0 mg Sodium

Acknowledgments

I USUALLY START OFF my acknowledgments by thanking my parents for their love and support but, Mom and Dad, you have moved your way up to the dedication page this time, so it's time for me to acknowledge my pint-sized ghost writer first this time. That ghost writer is none other than my precious daughter, Bradley. As I write these thank-yous and acknowledgments, I am eight months pregnant, but by the time this book is released you will be born and no doubt running the entire house. You have dictated every recipe in this book, from the seventeen weeks when I was too sick to cook or eat to the cravings for foods like One-Pot Jambalaya and Moon Dusted Donuts, which would have never made it into the book had I not been obsessing about them for weeks. My love for you has no words or limits. Thank you for keeping the book-writing process exciting, to say the least.

Thank you to Matthew Lore and the phenomenal team at The Experiment for being so endlessly kind, gracious, and supportive of me through the process of writing my third cookbook. It's always a rollercoaster ride, and this one seemed like it would never end. But here we are, with another finished book in hand, and I couldn't be more thrilled for the opportunity you have given me to share relatable, easy, fun, quick, and most important, vegan recipes.

Big thanks to Sara Lynn Paige not only for her breathtaking food photos but also for putting up with a scatter-brained pregnant girl with way too many things going on at once! You are truly amazing and wonderfully talented, and I look forward to working with you again.

Thank you to my awesome testers for trying nearly every recipe I put in front of you, giving me your honest feedback, and making me laugh along the way. You make the process of cookbook writing so fantastically fun. Thank you to Jessica

Berndt, Carrie Lynn Morse, Raelene Coburn, Celia Ozereko, Sherrie Thompson, Kelly Cavalier, Rachel Hallows, Constanze Reichardt, Tracy "The Vegan Butcher" Butcher, and Alee Vestal-Laborde.

Finally, thank you to you—yep, YOU! Thank you for picking up this book, thumbing through it, and giving it a try. To my readers who have been with me from my very first book, words can never express my gratitude to you. I hope I have continued to make you proud with this third book and that you love it just as much, if not more than, my first two. It has been such a pleasure to cook and create recipes for you over the past three years, and I look forward to continuing to do so for years to come!

About the Author

Alicia C. Simpson has been cooking since she was tall enough to reach the stove. She is the author of *Quick and Easy Vegan Comfort Food* and *Quick and Easy Vegan Celebrations* and the creator of the popular blogs Vegan Guinea Pig and The Lady and Seitan. She lives in Atlanta.